FLEXIBILITY
AND
BALANCE FOR
SENIORS

Secrets to Maintaining Movement and Strength

NICK & NORA ZANE

TABLE OF CONTENTS

Introduction 1

Chapter 1: Understanding Age-Related Physical Changes 5

The Science of Aging..8
Should I aim to Improve my Biological Age? 11
What Are Common Health Issues for Seniors? 13
The Psychological Impact...16

Chapter 2: The Fundamentals of Flexibility.................................19

Understanding Flexibility as a Senior 19
Types of Flexibility: How to Improve and Practice?...................21

Chapter 3: The Importance of Exercise and Cultivating Balance......37

Why Should I Exercise?..37
Will Exercise Make Me Fall? 39
What Is the Difference Between a Daily Workout and Daily Stretching? 40
What Kinds of Workouts Should I Do? 40
The Importance of Balance 41
How to Set Realistic Goals...46
What Happens if My Goals Fail? 53

Chapter 4: Getting Started: The Basics 55

How to Create a Safe Environment 56
Trust Your Mind-Body Connection: Be Mindful 59
Understanding Nutrition..67
A Note on Resilience..69

Chapter 5: Flexibility Exercises for Seniors 73

Stretching Essentials 73

What Are The Best Warm-Up And Stretching Strategies? 75

Why Should I Focus on My Form? 80

Chapter 6: Yoga 85

How Does One Go About Beginning A Yoga Journey? 87

Breathing Techniques: Yogic Breathing 93

Chapter 7: Tai Chi: The Art of Movement 99

What Are The Five Types of Tai Chi? 101

What Is The Aim of Tai Chi? 103

Chapter 8: Strength Training: A Pillar of Stability 105

Is Strength Training Safe for Seniors? 106

Can Strength Training Help with Sarcopenia or Osteoporosis? 106

Chapter 9: Motivation And Overcoming Challenges 111

Benefits of Motivation 112

How Can I Improve My Motivation? 112

What Happens if I Lose Motivation? 113

How to Overcome Challenges 115

Chapter 10: Movement Into Daily Life 119

Active Living Tips 121

Travel Adventures 122

Trusting Yourself 128

Conclusion: Evoking Joy 133

References 139

INTRODUCTION

Do you believe in aging gracefully? Take a minute and think about it. There's quite a bit of controversy surrounding the debate of whether or not age is just a number. Age is much more than a number, it's more of a representative of two important factors. The first is known as your chronological age and the other is known as your biological age. Your chronological age is determined by your actual age or how long you have been alive, while biological age is defined by the age of your cells. Here's the interesting thing about these two concepts of age: They don't represent the same age or number.

Fascinating, right? Of course, the fact that your body and its biology differ in age is incredible, it means that your biological age could be younger than your chronological age. Maybe, you've observed certain people around your age move through life without a stumble, stagger, or fall, exhibiting such incredible agility that you can't help but find yourself lodged between feelings of awe and envy. This is a completely normal response to have, there's nothing more frustrating than watching other people age with grace and ease. There are various reasons why certain people are successfully aging at a slower pace and this ultimately comes down to your brain health and overall lifestyle.

Now, you are probably thinking that brain health is not an essential topic to discuss since people aged fifty and beyond are prone to cognitive decline. This is true, but a common misconception about aging is that the issues—the decline in health—are normal and that it's normal for a person fifty years and older to stumble and fall due to age. This is because of the balance disorders that seniors are susceptible to, and though it is normal for many of us, with proper fitness goals we can improve and lower the risk of falling. This is where chronological and biological age comes in, when someone has a biological age that is lower than their chronological age—meaning that their body age is younger than their age in years—it is usually due to positive lifestyle choices that they accumulated throughout their lifespan.

Positive lifestyle choices can include a consistent and healthy diet and fitness routine, the influence of hobbies, and the dedication to constantly learning new skills. Our biological age will slow down when our overall health is balanced and continually promoted with stimulating challenges. What if you haven't been as active or mentally stimulated in your youth—don't beat yourself up about this, each of our lives tends to produce different results—is it still possible to slow down your biological age? Yes, it's still possible; however, it is still important to be realistic. Remember that you can't physically stop aging nor are there medication or nutrients available to reverse the effects of aging. Your goal—we will break down the positive effects of goals in a later chapter—should be to improve the overall quality of your life with better or healthier choices.

Once we hit the age milestone of fifty it's easy to understand and believe that life is strangely short; after all most of us have spent our former years parenting, nurturing a career, or simply trying to do our best, so it's strange to consider that it's never too late to re-evaluate what is important to you. As much as this book is about improving your fitness level, your flexibility, and reducing the risk of falling, we will also discuss a series of other vital factors required to improve the quality of your life and some practical steps on how you can develop these. Health is only one pillar of self-care, a practice, and an essential skill that can help you guarantee success throughout your life. We'll discuss the *practice* of self-care in more detail in a later chapter, but for now, let's look at the pillars of self-care. If I told you that there were five pillars within self-care, one focusing on health, what would the other pillars be for you?

Each pillar is designed to focus on a specific need, take health for example, within this pillar you are following sustainable practices to ensure that your overall health is functioning well. This allows you to construct goals and boundaries related to your health, from fifty onwards we're prone to declining health so to reach optimal health, you need to take steps to ensure that you follow a healthy diet and take into consideration any diseases or illnesses you have or might be prone to genetically. The goal is to make sure that you are prioritizing what is important to you. However, due to personal preference, our priorities and self-care practice won't be the same. Here are some examples of self-care pillars:

- Beauty
- Diet
- Love
- Career
- Travel
- Sleep
- Fitness
- Relationships
- Success
- Mental Health
- Spirituality

The list goes on, but the goal should be to choose the ones that are important to your well-being and future success. Alongside self-care, we'll discuss the positive benefits of mindfulness and how to create a positive outlook on life. We'll address the concept of aging from a realistic point of view, meaning that certain goals may be out of bounds—this is why it's important to have a good relationship with acknowledgment and acceptance. We'll get practical and discuss the positive influence fitness has on our lives, whether it's through yoga, tai chi, or strength training, and how continual practice will benefit your overall health.

Chapter 1:
UNDERSTANDING AGE-RELATED PHYSICAL CHANGES

Aging is a natural process that includes a series of physiological changes we endure throughout our lifespan. In some way, we're prepared to expect that major life changes will force us to reconstruct our lives. It is not the best of news, in fact, the idea of having to re-evaluate life as a senior might even feel unnecessary. However, I'm sure you've noticed aches taking effect in new spots, the sensation of loneliness becoming more consistent, or perhaps you noticed that your mobility is often hindered by moments where you've almost fallen. Regardless of what form of change your currently experiencing, as seniors, we are unfortunately forced to endure a constant change in our overall health. This change is not only in our physical health but our brain and mental health will continue to decline as well. However, take comfort in the fact that regardless of your age the presence of change will always be uncomfortable.

So, are there any preventive methods to limit or reduce the effect of change that comes with aging? No, it is best to acknowledge and accept that despite the discomfort lodged within this experience you have to face it. Acknowledgment goes a long way, being upfront about what is happening will allow us to move forward with positivity. If all you're going to do is sit and dwell, you'll only be holding yourself back and worsening most of the symptoms you're facing. This induces feelings of fear and anxiety—do you find yourself worrying about what you'll be like as you continue to age? These are normal and warranted concerns and I encourage you to acknowledge how difficult and overwhelming aging can be.

According to researchers at Harvard Health, it is possible to not only adapt to change but also encourage healthy aging by "finding new things you enjoy, staying physically and socially active, and feeling connected to your community and loved ones." (Smith et al., 2023, para.1). However, as with all change, the mere prospect of aging can bring feelings of fear and anxiety. Perhaps you've already experienced this type of age-related anxiety. Do you find yourself sometimes worrying about what you'll be like as you continue to age? About your family and about dealing with different types of loss? These arc normal and warranted concerns and I encourage you to acknowledge them, aging can be difficult and overwhelming. However, keep in mind that it is possible to reduce this fear and anxiety. The goal is to work towards maintaining and sustaining your physical, mental, and emotional health. This can be tricky, however, when we're told that it is not possible to sustain your health as you age. Here are three myths often associated with <u>aging:</u>

> ### <u>**MYTH**</u>
> **Aging means that my health has officially declined and that I'm now prone to disability.**
>
> ### <u>**FACT**</u>
> Not exactly, remember that aging is natural and that even children are going through the process. Aging doesn't necessitate negative health; however, as we enter our fifties, we become more prone to certain

diseases. Remember, just because you're getting older doesn't mean that you're automatically lodged into poor health or that you're going to be confined to a wheelchair or bed rest. Many seniors still live active and healthy lives by maintaining good overall health through fitness and diet.

MYTH
Getting older means that I'm going to lose my memories.

FACT
Eventually, we all lose some of our memory, and along the way, you'll find that it is harder to remember certain things. This is unfortunately inevitable but is a natural, albeit negative, effect on aging. However, by constantly seeking stimulating activity you can keep your brain active and sharp. So, don't be discouraged by memory loss.

MYTH
Getting older prohibits me from learning new skills.

FACT
No, it does not. Yes, your cognitive abilities might start to decline, and certain brain health conditions do become more prominent with age. However, we can help maintain our cognitive abilities by urgently treating specific conditions and keeping our brains stimulated. There are various skills to learn or activities that can help keep our brains active. Pursuing hobbies and staying physically active also helps support our brain health.

The Science of Aging

There are two fundamental types of aging, namely intrinsic and extrinsic aging.

Intrinsic Aging

This type of aging is also known as chronological aging and is ultimately determined by your genetic makeup; this means that each of us goes through processes differently and exhibits different symptoms of aging. This type of aging is affected by the body's ability to repair damage and deal with the degenerative effect of free radicals. Free radicals are defined as unstable molecules that damage various parts of your body (Elridge, 2022, para. 1). To keep free radicals in check we require sufficient levels of antioxidants in our system. Our bodies create free radicals, but they can also enter our systems through external sources. Free radicals are known to increase due to:

- environmental pollutants
- certain drugs and pesticides
- industrial solvents
- ultraviolet radiation like direct sunlight or tanning beds (Cleveland Clinic, 2022)

There are multiple reasons for intrinsic aging to occur—in addition to it being a natural process—here are some causes:

- Free radicals will damage your DNA and affect your skin's collagen and elastin structure.
- Hormonal changes, especially those induced by aging.

- Cell performance and decline due to your body's lack of capability to repair itself.

Intrinsic aging is natural and the Cleveland Clinic suggests that you consider it "as aging from the inside out" (2022, para.5).

Extrinsic Aging

This type of aging is also known as biological aging and is determined by the external factors in your life, whether it is the environment you're in or your lifestyle. The stress and pressures induced by your environment—whether it is toxic or loving—therefore affect how you age. The same goes for your nutrition and fitness regime. Here are some continuing factors that cause extrinsic aging:

- sun exposure
- smoking
- pollution
- chronic stress
- a lack of sleep and poor sleeping positions
- an unhealthy diet
- a lack of exercise (Esthetic Center, n.d.)

One thing to remember is that extrinsic aging negatively affects intrinsic aging by speeding up its process. Though both processes are natural, opting for healthier dietary and lifestyle choices can help slow down these processes. Factors that affect your extrinsic aging:

- air pollution
- tobacco smoke

- alcohol consumption
- malnutrition
- ultraviolet radiation exposure or UV exposure

Cellular Changes During Aging

Cells are often referred to as building blocks within the body, they are complex and provide structure to the body. One of their most important roles is to absorb nutrients from foods and convert them into energy for the body while carrying out other important functions. Cells are found in all living organisms and there are about thirty trillion of them performing various roles (MedlinePlus, 2021). There are over 200 hundred different cell types, and here are four you may recognize:

- red blood cells (also known as erythrocytes)
- skin cells
- neurons (also known as your nerve cells)
- fat cells

According to Cafasso, "Each of the 200 different types of cells in the body has a different structure, size, shape, and function" (2018, para.2). Our cells are in charge of making sure that our body remains effective. As we age, cells continue to lose their function, ultimately resulting in their death—this is the normal functioning of the body and a programmed process, meaning that your body not only expects this to happen but relies on it. The process is called apoptosis and is often referred to as cell suicide (Stefannaci, 2022)—rather dismal, right? Well, older cells must die for new cells to grow. Cells die for various reasons, and though some of these causes are natural, some are due to environmental influences.

Society and the media often encourage us to purchase items to restore cell growth or source items to prevent cell death. So, if you're interested in treating the skin itself, it is okay to source decent skin products and nutrition to help you. However, keep in mind that cells often die, not just because new ones need to grow, but because cells are unique, which means there is a limitation to the number of times they can divide and regrow—again, this limitation is decided by your genetic make-up. However, another reason why cells can get severely damaged is due to harmful substances, specifically treatments like radiation or chemotherapy.

Tips on How to Age Well

- Learn to cope with change, this is ultimately about building trust within yourself.
- Find meaning and live with joy, when we understand our ultimate purpose, we become more confident.
- Stay connected; make sure to always prioritize your relationships.
- Keep active and boost your vitality, even if it means going for a walk or doing some light stretching, the smallest amount of effort has an impact.
- Stay sharp, never stop educating yourself.

Should I aim to Improve my Biological Age?

This is a question people often ask when they learn about the different types of aging. However, note that one specific type of aging isn't necessarily better than the other. The two are interconnected and can function extremely well if we care for and maintain them equally. The most impressionable aspect about our biological age is that it supposedly keeps us young and mobile, and even though there is some truth in this, do remember that the goal is to maintain overall health.

How to Improve Your Biological Age

- Eat better: Nutrition is extremely important as we age, so focus on consuming foods that are high in nutrient quality and whole food. It may be an old-fashioned expression to eat the rainbow, but this is true, try to fill your plate as colorfully as you can and be mindful about the foods you're consuming.
  - Choose foods like fruits and vegetables, whole grains, and healthy fats (avocado oils and omega-3s).
  - Try to cut back on salt and alcohol, and avoid added sugars.
- Be more active: Since the overall goal is flexibility and stretching, try to begin with once a week to get a feel for the process. Next, try to incorporate practice for two to three days a week. Moderate to high-intensity training can be well managed throughout the week.
- Stop smoking if you're a smoker.
- Schedule your sleep and stick to a routine, remember that sleep allows the body and brain to initiate repair, and this ultimately improves your brain health.
- Be mindful of your weight and everything you're consuming, remember that your bone density starts to decrease once you reach 50, so infusing more calcium into your system will ultimately improve your overall health.

- Management: Always check in with your:
  - blood sugar levels
  - blood pressure
  - cholesterol levels

What Are Common Health Issues for Seniors?

According to Vann, "Once you make it to 65, the data suggest that you can live another 19.3 years, on average, according to the Centers for Disease Control and Prevention (CDC)" (2016, para.1). There are various ways to stay healthy, for example, by reducing unhealthy lifestyle choices like smoking or by losing a bit of weight. However, you must be strict and consistent, and include physical activity alongside a healthy diet. The first step you need to take to get ahead of things is a chat with your medical practitioner, the most common conflicts that hinder better health for us are common health issues. It is recommended to chat with your medical practitioner if you have any current health concerns and do a full medical check-up to see whether you should prepare for any other concerns in the future. Let's look at some common health issues affecting seniors

Common Health Issues Among Seniors

Arthritis

Arthritis is a type of inflammation pain that affects the joints, causes stiffness, and worsens with age. This is the most common health issue among people over 65 (Vann, 2016). It is easy to become discouraged when battling with arthritis; however, a personalized action plan can help you succeed. Here are some tips to help you manage when you suffer from arthritis:

- Keep moving, remember to stretch every day.
- Be mindful of your posture.
- Respect your limits, arthritis will limit you.
- Manage your weight with activity and a healthy diet.
- Quit smoking if you haven't already.

Heart Disease

Heart disease refers to a series of conditions that affect the heart, one of the more common types of heart disease is coronary artery disease (CAD) which affects the flow of blood toward the heart. As we age, our chances of developing heart disease increase, mainly due to an increase in blood pressure and cholesterol levels that can eventually lead to a stroke (Vann, 2016). As with your overall health, including physical activity and nutrition can provide numerous benefits to your heart health. Some additional tips include:

- Stop smoking and cut your alcohol consumption—if you engage in either of these.
- Work on your sleep hygiene, including your hours and quality of sleep.
- Be mindful of your blood pressure, cholesterol levels, and blood sugar levels.
- Consult your medical practitioner about possible medications to aid your health.

Cancer

Cancer is a disease that allows for a group of abnormal cells to split and damage your body tissue. Cancer is the second leading cause of death for people over the age of 65 (Vann, 2016). Due to the numerous measures available to detect cancer cells early, many cancers are treatable. Although cancer is not always preventable or treatable, treatments have improved significantly, and by detecting it early, following the advice of your healthcare professional, and maintaining a healthy lifestyle, you can improve your quality of life as a senior living with cancer (Vann, 2016).

Respiratory Disease

Chronic respiratory diseases are a collection of disorders such as asthma, cystic fibrosis, emphysema, and lung cancer. These diseases are considered to be the third most common causes of death among people 65 and older (Vann, 2016). These diseases are often manageable with tests and medication; however, paired with a good diet and physical activity offer even more benefits.

Alzheimer's Disease

Alzheimer's disease, which eventually turns into dementia, is a disease that progressively affects our mental functions, like memory. This disease is extremely common among older people and symptoms begin early in life. Vann states that "it's difficult to know exactly how many people are living with this chronic condition. Still, experts acknowledge that cognitive impairment has a significant impact on senior health across the spectrum," (n.d., para.6).

Once diagnosed with Alzheimer's, there are various management tips to help ease the transition:

- stay active.
- stimulate your mind with activity.
- rest and work on good sleep hygiene.

Osteoporosis

This is a medical condition that affects the bones, allowing them to become fragile and brittle due to loss of tissue. "Osteoporosis can contribute to becoming less mobile and potentially disabled should you fall and have a fracture or as the vertebral bodies collapse," (Vann, n.d., para.7).

The Psychological Impact

Aging ultimately leads to a significant change in many physiological factors, and as we continue to age one of the more common emotional and mental issues, we face is loneliness. Here, there is one point we need to clarify: Loneliness and aloneness are not the same. Aloneness is an intentional choice and serves to protect the individual's sense of self-awareness. Loneliness often occurs in old age and exasperates feelings of abandonment and burden. Often, at this stage in our lives, the consistency of change and illness can seemingly convince us that we've become a burn to those around us. Along with the change in our bodies is the presence of limitations and the unfortunate realization that we're forced to miss important, and not-so-important, social events and engagements due to declining health. In addition, these are some of the psychosocial problems we can develop with aging (Physio-pedia, n.d.):

- poor adjustment to role changes
- poor adjustment to lifestyle changes
- family relationship problems
- grief
- low self-esteem
- anxiety and depression
- aggressive behavior

There are various risk factors associated with physiological issues, just because you're older doesn't mean that the stressors others continue to face in their life will dissipate from yours. "Older adults may experience reduced mobility, chronic pain, frailty, diabetes, hearing loss, osteoarthritis or other health problems, all requiring some form of long-term care" (Physio-pedia, n.d., para.3). Mental health has an extraordinary impact on physical health, while physical health, in return, also has an impact on mental health—this is referred to as the mind and body connection and we'll get into discussing it in chapter 4. However, ultimately, we must aim to protect our mental health throughout this journey since aging will always be a new experience and often a strange process.

Chapter 2:
THE FUNDAMENTALS OF FLEXIBILITY

According to the Merriam-Webster (2023) dictionary, being flexible is "characterized by a ready capability to adapt to new, different, or changing requirements." However, a more modern and commonly used definition of flexibility refers to a person being able to bend into various positions and poses easily. The act of flexibility is often associated with particular athletes and dancers seeking to improve their form, gymnasts and ballet dancers are specifically known for their flexibility, and their ability is often idolized as a fitness goal. However, flexibility doesn't only relate to athletes or dancers, it extends to everyone and has become specifically important in seniors' health practices. Due to the decline in motion and balance, and the risk of falling, seniors require flexibility to minimize the possibility of any significant damage. The series of stretches outlined in this section can help with increasing our range of motion and improving our flexibility.

Understanding Flexibility as a Senior

The reality for us senior citizens is that our physical health decreases in the range of accessibility. This means that our muscles and joints stiffen with age and affect the durability of our motion. Again, this may seem like an inevitable part of old age; however, the practice of flexibility isn't aimed as a preventive measure or a cure. Flexibility in old age is instead about the sustainability of motion. Yes, indeed, flexibility is often dismissed as a practice that only helps to locate or reduce stress, and certain yoga postures not only make you aware of stiffness or a lack of range in your muscles and joints but also help you pinpoint exactly where stress is located—but we'll discuss this a bit later. Flexibility is more than just the body's ability to bend, when we can successfully increase the range of motion within our muscles and joints, our joints can extend beyond their original capability, and we become more agile. The ultimate aim of flexibility is to promote healthy movement.

What Is Healthy Movement?

We achieve healthy movement when our muscles and joints can successfully and effectively complete daily movements without any restriction or pain. To achieve this, we need to regularly practice stretches and routines that promote flexibility. By improving flexibility and healthy movement, our muscles can coordinate between themselves, putting less strain and pressure on the rest of the body. Healthy movement helps you feel physically and emotionally, helps secure your productivity levels, and improves your cognitive abilities.

The Benefits of Flexibility

Improving your flexibility offers a wide range of benefits:

- By developing your range of motion, your risk of injury will decrease. This helps to reduce the likelihood of muscular or joint injuries that seniors are prone to, such as stiffness in joints, arthritis, fatigue, weakness, muscle tension, and risk of falling.

- Your stress levels will reduce the more you stretch, and your serotonin levels (your feel-good hormone) will boost your mood, lowering your risk of depression and anxiety.
- It will enhance your agility and increase your range of movement, allowing you to move more freely and easily throughout your day.
- You'll be able to recover from pain more effectively.
- You'll notice an improvement in your ability to complete daily tasks.
- Your muscles will endure an increase in blood flow.
- You'll experience less pain or a reduction in your pain levels.
- It will improve your overall physical performance in a range of activities.
- It will help you secure a more positive mindset.

Types of Flexibility: How to Improve and Practice?

When it comes to practicing flexibility, it is important to first understand the various types of flexibility practices there are to follow. Four important types of stretching affect your range of motion and can ultimately increase your flexibility levels if you engage with them through consistent practice. Let's look at these four types: active, passive, dynamic, and ballistic stretching.

Active Stretching

To activate the hamstring muscles. Easier said than done, right? You are allowed to use accessories like yoga straps or resistant bands. However, when you are able to hold the stretch without any assistance, your hip flexors and core muscles will activate to maintain the hold of the leg in the air and preserve the hamstring stretch.

Active stretching is a simple process, and we mostly rely on it to help with muscle recovery. Therefore, we often use active stretching after a workout as part of a recovery program and a way to decrease any potential muscle damage. For the same reason, these stretches are also a popular pre-workout warm-up. However, you incorporate these stretches in your workout routine, remember that what works for one person won't necessarily work for the next. The best advice that anyone could ever give to you in terms of health and fitness would be to listen to your body before making any permanent decisions. A great way to improve your active stretching techniques is through yoga, which we will discuss yoga in a later chapter—in fact, many of the stretches used here are also used in yoga practice. The only difference between the two is that yoga is about promoting fluid movement between each pose.

Since active stretching doesn't require equipment unless you need the assistance of a strap or resistance band, you can practice it anywhere and in any space you have available. Here's how to practice any active stretch:

- Decide on an area or muscle you want to stretch and choose a particular pose that targets that area.
- Flex the agonist muscles, remember that this is the same muscle on the opposite side of the muscle being stretched.
- Hold the position for about ten seconds depending on your capability, remember that gradual progress is vital. Don't rush anything.
- Once you have completed the stretch it is best to repeat the same stretch on the opposite side, or limb—if it is a bilateral stretch.

In the table below are four examples of active stretches with a more detailed approach to the muscle groups that they target. Keep in mind that the agonist is the muscle working and the antagonist is the muscle being stretched.

About the Stretch

- Benefit: the great thing about this stretch is its ability to reduce back pain, improve your posture, and prevent soreness and injury. This is due to the muscle's proximity to your spine and hip flexors.
  - Remember that you shouldn't be experiencing pain when you practice this stretch.
- Target: the hamstrings
- Agonist: the hip flexors and your core muscles
- Antagonist: the hamstrings
- Note: There are various forms of hamstring stretching; however, the lying hamstring stretch is always a great place for the beginner.
- How to (lying hamstring stretch):
  - Lie down flat on your back, if you feel you need a pillow for your neck you are more than welcome to add one. Bend both knees.
  - If you are using a strap apply it to the base of the foot that will be stretched, now raise the leg of the muscle that will be stretched. You will feel resistance to the accessory you are using, remember not to force anything.
  - Remember to activate your core and hip flexors, these muscles are used to secure your stability.
  - Hold the pose for ten to twenty seconds, if you are more advanced you are more than welcome to extend until thirty seconds.

- After the allocated time has passed, switch to the other leg and repeat this process at least three times per leg.

Advice: if you notice any sign of pain or discomfort within your lower back or tailbone, lower your leg at a slanted angle to prevent the presence of pain.

Active chest stretch

- Benefit: This stretch activates your chest muscles, forcing the chest to open up while stimulating blood flow. However, this stretch will also affect your auxiliary muscles encouraging your breathing muscles to work better.
- Target: the chest muscles (your pectoral muscles) and biceps
- Agonist: the deltoids, rhomboids, mid traps, and other back or shoulder-related muscles.
- Antagonist: the chest muscles and your biceps
- Note: In yoga, this stretch is often used and referred to as a heart opener.
- How to:
  - Stand up straight and stretch your arms out to your sides at a ninety-degree angle. Though you are keeping your arms straight, remember to maintain a slight bend in your elbow to protect the joint.
  - A tip to increase the intensity of this stretch would be to either open your palms and turn them up to the ceiling or face them straight forward.
  - Remember to open your arms as wide as possible, they must be extended from behind your body, and when you begin to feel a

stretch across your chest and the front of your arms, hold it for about ten to fifteen minutes.

Tip, hold your chest up and open, your rib cage should be flaring, and your back shouldn't be arching.

Active quad stretch

- Benefit: by stretching the quads regularly we're naturally increasing their range of mobility, flexibility, and the range of motion between the hip joints and the knee. When our quads are activated, they prohibit injury, and pain, and improve your posture.
- Target: the quadriceps
- Agonist: your hamstrings
- Antagonist: your quadriceps
- How to:
  - Stand tall and keep your feet at hip distance apart, try and maintain good posture with a slight bend in your knees to protect the joints and muscles. You can use a wall or chair for balance.
  - Start with your left leg, lift and bend the knee, moving the foot toward your butt.
  - Make sure that your lifted knee is pointing toward the floor while aligned with your standing knee.
  - Try to get the foot of your left leg closer to your butt, don't force the stretch, and hold it for ten to fifteen minutes.

Tip: if the knee moves forward, you will be flexing from your hips instead and this won't produce the same result, so be mindful of your posture.

Active triceps stretch

- Benefit: The stretch aims to help the muscle maintain a good range of motion after training, especially strength training. Stretches related to the triceps ease any form of tightness, not only in your triceps but also in your shoulders and back.
- Target: the triceps
- Agonist: the biceps and your shoulder muscles
- Antagonist: the triceps
- Note: There are several forms of this stretch for you to work through, we'll start with the overhead triceps stretch.
- How to (overhead triceps stretch):
    - Stand up straight and extend your left arm into the air, as if you are trying to touch the ceiling or sky.
    - Bend your left elbow so that your forearm and hand are lower behind your head and neck, settling between your shoulder blades.
    - Make sure that your elbow continues to point toward the sky, now using your right hand gently push the left elbow down. This will increase the range and intensity of the stretch.
    - Hold this stretch for about ten to fifteen seconds. Release your arm slowly and repeat the stretch a few times.
    - Repeat the stretch on the other side.

Passive Stretching

Passive stretching, on the other hand, is about staying in one position throughout the stretch while relying on an accessory to hold and maintain the stretch. Due to the static structure of the stretch, it might look easy, but we often overestimate our body's ability to stretch, so always take the stretches slowly and listen to your body. Passive stretching is a static form of stretching that after you enter the stretch, you deepen into it—as deep and comfortable as you can reach. When you reach a place of tension, you then hold the stretch with the help of the accessory for about a minute. Here's what to remember: Your place of tension and how deep you can stretch will determine your limit, do not push past this limit. With consistent practice, you'll be able to improve how deep you can take the stretch if you overdo it at the start, you risk injuring yourself. The ultimate point of this type of stretch is to allow your body to relax, which you can achieve by stretching up to your point of tension (or limit) and then slowly releasing and relaxing your muscles making sure to not force or hurt yourself. An example of this stretch is the supine single-leg stretch, which is a great one to begin with because you don't need an accessory or much help.

Here is how to do the supine single-leg stretch:

- Lie down on your back with your legs straight and stretched out, find a comfortable position, and be mindful of your breathing.
- Raise your left leg straight into the air, it is okay to keep a slight bend in the knee to protect the joint. Keep the right leg straight on the ground.
- Either interlace your hands around your left thigh or place a strap or a towel around the bottom of your foot. The aim is to pull your leg toward you while the resistance of the strap, towel, or hands serve as resistance.

- Hold this pose for about a minute and then gently release the leg and repeat on the opposite side.

Passive stretching requires care, especially if you are new to the stretch, you could injure a muscle. Passive stretching shouldn't hurt, it is about trusting and listening to your body. Whenever you feel any sense of pain, make sure to release the stretch slowly, and first check for any muscle tension before continuing.

In the table below are two examples of passive stretches with detailed steps of how to perform each stretch. Remember to take your time whenever you are attempting a new stretch, make sure you know exactly which movement to do and in what order. If you are ever stuck, take a breath and then slowly release the stretch before you look at the instructions again.

Butterfly stretch

This stretch has numerous modifications and is commonly found in yoga.

- Begin seated on the floor with the soles of your feet pressing into each other. You can deepen the intensity of the stretch by moving your legs closer to your hips. However, if it causes pain, don't force intensity and keep them as near as possible.
- Solidify your legs and sitting bones, lengthen your spine, and fold over your legs.
- Remember to breathe as you lengthen your spine and stop where you are comfortable.
- Hold the pose for thirty seconds, improving gradually with duration.
- Repeat two to four times.

The forward fold stretch

This stretch is also common in yoga and serves as a hamstring stretch.

- Seated on the ground with your legs extended, sit up straight, and be mindful of your hips and knees—keep a slight bend in them to protect the joint.
- Inhale deeply and begin to fold forward, reaching your hands toward your toes.
- Remember to bend from your hips and not your lower back, this stretch shouldn't hurt and if there is pain in your back, stop. Also, if you can't reach your toes, reach only as far as you can.
- Hold the stretch for thirty seconds as you begin.

Repeat two to four more times.

Dynamic Stretching

Dynamic stretching is also known as a dynamic warm-up and is an extremely popular warm-up routine because it targets muscle groups strategically. These types of stretches are focused, controlled, and specific. The best time to use dynamic stretching is with a strength and weight-based workout.

The Difference Between Dynamic and Static Stretches

Why is it important to differentiate the two forms of stretching? For starters both forms of stretching offer completely different results and can be strategically used in specific fitness routines.

Dynamic Stretching Defined

- More commonly used in exercise practices and sports-related activities.
- A more energetic approach is used to prepare the body for a particular physical activity, targeting a specific amount or group of muscles.
- This stretching uses a repetition of specific exercises targeting muscles repetitively to improve your performance within each muscle group.
- Remember that we usually rely on this form of stretching to prepare for physical activity, as in a warm-up.
- A rep count will be used; this means that you may repeat the same stretch for a specific number of times and sets.
- This form of stretching focuses on specific stretches that help increase muscle mobility and usage for the intended sport. Note, that swimmers and hockey players may use different stretches to increase their physical activity but might still follow the same pattern of sequence.

Static Stretching Defined

- This form of stretching is also used in a variety of sports-related activities.
- A slower approach is used to control the movement, specifically after completing an exercise or workout.
- This stretching practice requires you to repeat a specific stretch in a slow and controlled manner to slow down the muscle groups that you have used, preparing the muscles for rest.
- Remember that we mostly rely on this form of stretching to cool down from a physical activity.
- This stretch focuses on holding the stretch for a limited amount of time.

- This form is mainly focused on preparing the body and its muscles used for rest and ultimately for repair.

When is The Best Time to Use Dynamic Stretching?

Well, preferably before a workout or a specific sports activity.

- Before sports or athletics: According to studies focused on dynamic stretching and sports, these stretches have extremely beneficial performance results for those taking part in sports such as running, jumping, basketball, soccer, and sprint racing (Chertoff, 2019).
- Before weightlifting: This will further improve the range of power and extension needed for the workout.
- Before cardiovascular exercises: It is a great resource to warm up your muscles and joints and will reduce the risk of injury and improve performance.

Below are four examples of dynamic stretches that target the hips, arms, and leg muscles.

Dynamic Stretches

Hip circles

- You can use the counter, a wall, or a chair for support.
- Stand with your feet hip-width apart, then lift your left leg, keeping it bent, and gently open or swing it to the side.
- Do twenty circles on one leg and then switch to the other leg. This is good for hip flexors.

Arm circles

- Stand with your feet hip-width apart and open up your arms to the sides, keeping a slight bend in the elbow.
- Keep your palms facing down while they're hovering at shoulder height.
- Slowly move your arms in circles going forward twenty times, before reversing the direction. The aim is not to drop your arms during this movement.

Lunge and twist

- Stand with your feet together, with your left leg take a big step forward—if you require support use a wall or table—and stabilize that left foot as it presses down with your hip and knee gently begin to bend.
- Lower down in the lunge, hovering your right knee above the ground, balancing on the right foot—only go as far as your flexibility allows.
- Keep your torso upright and as you press into your left knee, make sure not to extend it beyond your left toes.
- While your right leg hovers, fold your hands into a prayer position keeping them pressed against your chest as you turn your upper body toward the left. There are other variations of this part, but this is the basic move to start with.
- Slowly release and swing back around, rise up a bit, and step forward.
- Repeat this movement on the other leg by stepping back with your right leg.

Squat and leg lift

- Stand with your feet hip-width apart and with your toes pointing outwards, your arms are fine wherever they're comfortable.

- Lower down into a squat, or a half squat if you are more comfortable.
- As you rise back up, press your weight into your left leg. Lift your right leg sideways with your inner thigh parallel to the floor.
- As you return this leg back to formation, prepare yourself for another squat, and as you rise up this time lift the left leg.
- Repeat this movement 10-12 times on each side.

Ballistic Stretching

Ballistic stretching shares similarities with the stretches usually used to warm up, it is used across all types of physical activity. It is known as an intense stretching practice that often requires a series of bouncing movements to exert the body beyond its normal range of motion. One of the major differences it has to passive stretching is that ballistic stretching focuses on stretching muscles at a quicker pace. For example, the ballistic stretching version of touching your toes will have you adding a bouncing movement as you touch your toes. Ballistic stretching isn't for everyone, meaning that if your medical practitioner suggests that you avoid this method for the sake of your health, it is perfectly fine since there are three other methods to try.

However, an important thing to understand about the usage of "bounces", which is commonly used in ballistic stretching is that it refers to "pulsing" or "pulses" instead of jerking or interrupted movements. The most common reason people fail at ballistic stretching is that it is often performed incorrectly. There are numerous benefits to ballistic stretching including:

- an increase in flexibility
- higher levels of capability and endurance
- an improvement in your tendon elasticity

- a reduction in muscle soreness
- improved blood circulation
- reduced levels of fatigue
- enhanced motor skills

Below are four examples of some ballistic stretches. Remember that with ballistic stretches the aim is to use pulses as you move but if you are new to the stretch, take it slow, listen to your body, and go at your own pace.

Ballistic Pancake

- Sit on the ground with your legs spread as far apart as possible.
- The goal is to lean forward and bend from the hips and not the lower back—be mindful of this.
- Start bending from the hips and pull your chest flat toward the ground.
- Stretch as far as you can and don't force the movement.
- Sit back up and repeat the stretch.
- Move in a way that feels natural to you, you can even incorporate a flow or rhythm to your movement.

Ballistic toe touch

- Stand tall, with your feet together, and a slight bend in your knees to protect the joints.
- On an inhale, stretch your arms toward the sky as far as you can reach.
- Exhale and reach down toward your toes, go as far as you can, and remember that bend in your knees.

- Inhale and move your hands back up towards the sky. Make sure not to rise too quickly. If you feel faint as your blood rushes from your head, take a moment.
- Repeat the stretch. As your hands reach up to the sky, incorporate a small bounce in between each stretch.

Ballistic core twist

- Stand tall with your feet hip distance apart, extend your arms to your side, and engage your core. Remember that you will be twisting from your core, so keep it engaged.
- Twist your torso to the left and back to the center, then move on and twist to the right side.
- Feel free to swing your arms as you move, if you feel like it.

Ballistic runner stretch

- Begin in a runner's lunge. This stretch mimics the lunge but requires you to lengthen your front leg and keep it on its heel.
- Fold forward from the hips and reach for your toes—reach as far as you can.
- Once you reach the bottom or near enough, begin to perform your bounces.
- Move back up and repeat on the other side.

Ballistic hurdle stretch

- Sit on the ground with your left leg extended out in front of you and the right foot bent behind you at a ninety-degree angle.

- Once comfortable in the stretch, reach both arms over your extended leg, aiming for the outside of the left leg.
- Perform your bounces, before switching legs.

Ballistic standing offset toe touch

This stretch is very similar to toe touches, the key difference being that one foot will be in front of the other which will allow tension on the back leg, in the hamstrings. In this position, you will perform your bounces before switching feet.

Chapter 3:
THE IMPORTANCE OF EXERCISE AND CULTIVATING BALANCE

Exercise is a physical activity that improves our physical and mental health and optimizes body function. Another interesting description of exercise is that it's a physical effort. In this case, *effort* may take months of practice before there is any evidence of progress. This is why resilience goes a long way. It stops you from giving up or feeling defeated which can affect your progress.

Why Should I Exercise?

Firstly, no one is ever too old to start something new, so exercise at fifty and beyond is not a big deal. The decision to start exercising and to keep on going is ultimately up to you, no one else can make it for you. When starting a new exercise routine, it is best to first discuss the health risks with your medical practitioner. They will also be able to give you advice about which types of exercises might be best for you, especially if you have any specific health conditions or concerns.

The Benefits of Exercise

Regular exercise has many physical, mental, and social benefits. Let's have a look at some of them.

- Physical benefits:
    - Helps you maintain or lose body weight.
    - Helps increase your metabolism.
    - Improves your balance.
    - Lowers blood pressure.
    - Reduces the risk of heart disease.
    - Increases muscle strength and function.
    - Reduces the risk of certain cancers.
    - Improves bone health and strength.
    - Lowers the risk of type 2 diabetes.
- Mental benefits:
    - Reduces the risk of mental health disorders.
    - Promotes positivity.
    - Reduces your stress levels.
    - Reduces the risk of Alzheimer's disease and dementia.
    - Improves your mood and overall wellbeing.
    - Helps increase your energy levels.
    - Helps improve your sleep quality.
- Social benefits:
    - Reduces feelings of loneliness.
    - It will improve your self-esteem and boost your confidence levels.
    - Helps make you more accountable and improves your discipline and health habits.

- ○ Helps increase your motivation levels and inspiration to succeed.
- ○ Improves your ability to set goals and accomplish them.
- ○ Increases your levels of empathy.
- ○ Helps improve your communication skills.
- ○ Helps you live a more balanced lifestyle.

Will Exercise Make Me Fall?

No. However, if you fall or stumble during a particular exercise, it is likely due to an accident or misstep. This is why mindful movement is extremely important. You shouldn't be rushing through your routine and rushing to improve the range or level of the exercise. Though older adults are prone to falls and injury, the risk of injury brought on by poor form can affect anyone. Patience goes a long way and so does resilience, exercise is about consistency and effort. Most of us lack these traits, but they can be improved upon with time—which in return will improve our cognitive abilities. Another important factor about exercising is stretching and warm-up, these are two separate and equally important practices. A healthy warm-up session before beginning any form of workout can also help prevent accidents or missteps. However, stretching is not only a form of warm-up or cool-down exercises, but it can also be practiced on its own and even daily.

What Is the Difference Between a Daily Workout and Daily Stretching?

The most significant difference is the rest and repair needed after and in between each of the practices. You don't have to necessarily enjoy stretching to do strength training, most people tend to choose a form of workout that they enjoy or fits with their lifestyle. However, there is more success in combining practices, for example, stretching will improve your range of mobility, allowing you to extend and lengthen your muscles through various exercises. You can practice stretching daily, especially light stretching on active rest days. However, for strength training to be effective it should be done around three days a week with rest scheduled in between sessions. Muscles need time to rest and repair—this restorative process takes place when we sleep which is why it is important to improve your overall sleep quality when you're engaging in strength training.

What Kinds of Workouts Should I Do?

The four main types of workouts are endurance, strength, balance, and flexibility training. The aim is to incorporate a combination of these practices in your workout routine to improve your health. Let's look at the four types a bit more closely.

- Endurance: This improves your ability to walk or run for extended periods and your overall ability to move.
    - Examples of this include cycling, seated volleyball, and walking.

- Strength: This not only allows you to build muscle but also helps your body maintain muscle mass. Strength training also helps to improve your balance.
  - You can use weights and resistance bands to improve and build muscle mass, though bodyweight exercises are also popular for seniors.
- Balance: This is about reducing your fall risk. You can improve your balance through a series of exercises and stretches.
  - This can be gained through stretches, yoga, and tai chi.
- Flexibility: This is mostly gained through yoga and stretching, flexibility isn't just focused on improving your ability to bend but also improving your ability to perform various other exercises.
  - Yoga is a safe way to achieve flexibility.

The Importance of Balance

Balance is the foundation of mobility and we're often unaware of its impact on our day-to-day lives or the many activities in which we find ourselves invested. Balance is important because it not only allows us to complete various tasks but also reduces the risk of falling. As older adults, we're made to believe that falling is an accepted part of our old age and that stumbling and staggering throughout life is inevitable. This is not true though. We can sustain good mobility throughout our lives. Age reduces muscle mass and our nerves become prone to stress which affects our reaction time, or reflexes. By engaging in balancing exercises, we can help improve our mobility and reduce the risk of falling.

Why Should You Improve Your Balance?

Well, for starters it is only going to worsen without care, but here are some reasons to improve your balance. Firstly, it helps to prevent injury, as aging adults we're prone to falls and with the aid of balance, we lower the risk of injury. Secondly, with balance, you're taking care of a group of muscles and allowing them to combine in practice to achieve ultimate release.

Will Balance Prevent Falls?

Yes, it will, because when we practice balance-strengthening exercises we're ultimately taking care of our core muscles and overall muscle mass. This means that with a strong core, we're able to endure more throughout our day.

What Are The Signs of Balance Problems in Seniors?

Despite the fact that falls are inevitable, some of us may experience the same symptoms in varying ranges of discomfort and pain. Here are some signs to look for,

- blurry vision
- periods of confusion
- diarrhea
- vertigo or dizziness
- nausea and vomiting
- fear, anxiety, or panic
- a sensation of falling
- fluctuations in heart rate and blood pressure
- feelings of lightheadedness, faintness, or floating (Madison, 2021)

What Causes Seniors to Fall?

Age is the most prominent determining factor for balance issues in seniors; however, there are several other reasons why a balance disorder may occur. The most common issue that causes issues with seniors' balance is inner ear problems. According to the Cleveland Clinic (2021, para. 2), "Labyrinthitis is an inner ear infection characterized by inflammation of the labyrinth. The labyrinth is the inner ear system responsible for your hearing and sense of balance." When the labyrinth or its nerves are inflamed, it severely affects balance and hearing. This is ultimately due to the brain struggling to make sense of the mismatched information it receives due to the inflammation. One of the common effects due to the pressure within the brain is vertigo which is characterized by feelings of dizziness and spinning.

Training to Improve Balance

Tightrope walk

For this exercise, you're going to need some string or tape that you place securely on a straight line on the floor.

- Start at one end and hold your arms out wide to the sides.
- Begin to walk without stepping off on the sides.
- Aim to do fifteen steps.

You can mix up this flow of stepping movement by stepping backward or interchanging each foot with each step.

Rock the boat

- Place your feet hip-width apart and distribute your weight equally on each side.
- Inhale as you shift your weight onto your left foot and exhale as lift your right foot forward and as high as you can, this depends on your overall balance.
- Hold for up to thirty seconds before returning the leg and switching to the other foot.

Do five to ten reps per leg.

Flamingo stand

Standing tall, you can use a chair, wall, or tabletop for support during this stretch.

- Shifting your weight to your left leg, lift and bend your right leg while you're balancing on your left leg.
- Maintain good posture by making sure that your spine, neck, and head are in one straight line.
- Hold this pose for about fifteen seconds before switching to the opposite leg.

Plank with elbows on a stability ball

For this stretch, you'll need a stability ball.

- Using the ball as a balancing device, firmly place your elbows on the ball and stretch out into a plank.

- It is going to feel unstable, and this is okay. The aim is to challenge your core and overall stability. To find stabilization, you're going to have to practice breathing mindfully and patiently.
- Once you're in a plank you can begin to draw small circles with the ball and move ten times in one direction before reversing the direction.
- You could also simply hold the stretch in a plank for about fifteen seconds.

Chair leg raises

This exercise requires the use of a chair and if you're able to you could use ankle weights.

- Sit on the chair and keep your spine straight, both of your feet should be placed directly under your knees.
- Inhale and slowly begin to lift your left leg and hold it up for a few seconds.
- Exhale and gradually lower it back down and repeat with the other leg.
- Do one to three sets of ten to twenty-second repetitions.

Banded triplanes toe tap

This exercise requires the use of a resistance band, note that there are various levels of resistance, and you should begin with the lowest resistance for optimal effect.

- Place the band around your lower thighs, just above your knees, and stand with your legs hip-width apart or just until you feel resistance in the band.
- Lower down into a high squat, engaging your core and hip muscles.

- Gently lift your left leg just a few inches from the ground and use the resistance of the band to tap your foot forward, to the side, and straight behind you.
- Do ten to twenty repetitions before moving over to the other leg.

Single leg cross-body punches

For this exercise, you'll need some weights, light weights are best suited for this movement.

- Hold the dumbbells in each hand and at chest height.
- Lower into a high squat and shift your weight equally into both feet.
- Punch the weights across your body, one at a time.
- Do one to three sets of ten to twenty repetitions.

How to Set Realistic Goals

Let's face reality, we're not getting any younger and our overall health has launched itself into a continuum of decline. However, since we already know this, the decline in health and change in health shouldn't frighten us anymore. Accepting change is a difficult reality for most of us and it is okay if it is taking you a little more time to come to terms with the changes that aging brings. However, applaud yourself for taking the steps to improve your health. This is why setting goals is extremely important regardless of age or whatever situation you're currently facing. The great aspect of goal setting is that it is not measured in size, which means that whether you have achieved a small or large goal, you can experience the sensation of achievement or accomplishment.

Another great way of thinking about goals is viewing them as part maintenance and part sustainability. Consider the goal we first made before officially starting this journey, the one-off promoting healthier life choices through the practice of flexibility. In this case, the goal is flexibility, and we aim to maintain—and ensure the prosperity of this goal—by infusing secondary goals to support the overall goal of flexibility. By pursuing additional forms of activity, like the practice of mindfulness, self-care, yoga, and nutrition, for example, we're not only promoting brain health but are also improving our flexibility. So, by continuing to incorporate various goals (related to the promotion of flexibility) into the main goal (of flexibility), we're maintaining the health of the overall (or main) goal.

Sustainability in this regard refers to sourcing healthy methods to ensure the future prosperity of your lifestyle. This is why enforcing goals throughout your life is extremely important, it not only holds you accountable but also promotes improvement in your cognitive abilities. So, introducing sustainable habits to our current lives ensures the success of flexibility and prohibits the risk of falling. Sustainable habits can be considered as daily stretches—though remember to check in with your body—practicing gratitude each day through journalling, practicing meditation, and sourcing more joyful experiences in life through the connections we have with people.

The Benefits of Setting Goals

Goal setting offers a range of benefits, including:

- It helps provide direction in your life.
- It helps you focus which improves your ability to engage in the practice of mindfulness.

- It boosts your levels of productivity, which improves your ability to practice stretching and other hobbies.

- It helps you to gain clarity, which is vital when making decisions, and ideally helps you focus on the importance of your health.

- You'll have more free time or rather more time to explore things that are important to you. Most of us tend to find ourselves consumed in the lives of others or on the internet. Being aware of the goals you're seeking to achieve helps you to make choices that are aligned with your goals and helps you prioritize what is important to you.

- It makes you accountable for the maintenance and sustainability of the goal, meaning that you only have yourself to blame—although this isn't about blaming—for not following your routine.

- Your decision-making skills improve simply due to the focus on goals and everything important to you. The truth is that at this point in your life—if you have kids, they're likely grown—you don't have anyone but yourself to be responsible for, so when you're focused on prioritizing your needs and wants many decisions related to others and you are simple.

- You have more control over your life.

- Your goals can help motivate you to constantly succeed. The great thing about accomplishing any goal is the mood-boosting sensations that are released.

- You become inspired to continue achieving goals.

Why Should Seniors Set Goals?

The main reason should be due to your health, especially your brain health. Activity is vital for your health as a senior, mainly because of the changes and challenges your body and brain will face throughout the aging process.

Constant, stimulating activity that challenges the mind promotes brain health and can enrich your life. Hobbies are always encouraged, and goal setting helps with these in the form of setting a goal to learn a new hobby or improve an existing skill.

Where Are Goals Set?

You can set goals in every aspect of your life, there isn't a correct or incorrect manner to set them, the only thing to remember is to be kind to yourself and realistic about the goals you're setting. Here are common areas where goalsetting can be quite useful:

- Health: These forms of goals are the most common when we start aging and realize the impact that our health has on our daily lives. Examples of these goals include weight loss, specific fitness goals, a healthier diet, or following the requirements of specific medical illnesses.
- Relationships: These goals focus on improving the connections we have with people and are vital to the health of seniors since the levels of loneliness increase as we age. Relationship goals often relate to spending more time with people you love.
- Financial: This is usually focused on reducing the amount of money we spend and thinking more logically about the future and retirement. As we age, downsizing becomes important to overall health simply because we won't have time to keep up with certain habits that were once important. And this is okay, make peace with the fact that certain factors in your life will have to be adapted. For example, maybe you were more active with your social outings, time will reduce the number of outings you'll be able to endure within a week.

- Learning: This is a great goal to have, especially as we age—we've already stressed the importance of challenging your cognitive abilities—constantly learning will aid these abilities and positively affect your brain health.

What Are SMART Goals?

The SMART goal strategy focuses on refining your expectations and ultimately becoming more conscious of what you want and expect from life. The great aspect of this strategy is that it can be used in every aspect of your life, meaning that you can apply this strategy to your relationship goals and then separately use it to determine what it is you want from those specific areas. The purpose of this system is to refine not only your expectations but also to help you discover what exactly you hope to achieve with the introduction of a new goal.

SMART goal strategies

SMART goals focus on specificity and determining exactly what it is you want. It is also a great tool to use to help determine what exactly your goal should be. Here are five important questions to answer, the "five W questions, which help you determine specific goals:

- What do I want to accomplish?
- Why is this goal important?
- Who is involved?
- Where is it located?
- Which resources or limits are involved? (Mind Tools, n.d.)

So, if your goal is to gain a promotion at work, perhaps you want to become a manager, here's how to effectively and specifically state this goal: I want to become the manager in my team and will need to improve and gain the necessary skills to succeed.

Measurable

This step is about being mindful of progress and motivation, a factor we commonly tend to struggle with when working toward a goal is the loss of motivation—we discuss motivation in more detail in Chapter 9. However, when we're motivated, we're able to fully comprehend our wants and desires, and critically think about what it is we need. Reflection is a great place to start, it is going to help you fully understand your goal and how to measure it.

Achievable

Setting achievable goals is about being realistic about the goals you want, remember that a lack of clarity will hinder the success of the goal. So, keep the goal within the realm of possibility. This isn't to say that you should minimize your goals, but your goal can't be to be a millionaire by retirement if you're close to retirement and haven't taken the necessary steps toward that goal. Every goal needs to be set within a specific timeframe, so if you want to achieve millionaire status by retirement be logical about the steps you need to achieve this status. The truth is that any goal is likely achievable with realism and hard work. According to Mind Tools (n.d., para. 4), these are the questions you must answer to set an achievable goal:

- What do I need to accomplish this goal?
- What skills do I need to achieve this goal?

- How realistic is this goal based on my overall lifestyle?
- How will this goal impact my financial life, what are the necessary steps (to improve) to take?

Relevant

Your goals need to be based on your life and who you are. Most of the time we find ourselves making mindless decisions about life, especially when we're not fully aware or accepting of our current situation. For example, as we age, we go through a series of body and health changes, which is a difficult process of change that can be challenging for many of us to accept. Although it is fine to take your time, you must keep in mind that if you haven't fully acknowledged or accepted your circumstance it is likely that your goals are going to suffer.

Here is a different way of looking at it, say that you have been following a specific diet (by choice) for years, but due to the decline in age and health concerns you have to change this diet and eat foods you have avoided for years. This can take a mental toll and could mean that your lifestyle and relevant goals aren't properly aligned. With aging, we need to make sure that the goals we're setting work with and change with our lifestyle. Relevant goals are determined by answering "yes" to these questions (Mind Tools, n.d., para.6.):

- Is this worthwhile?
- Is it the right time to set this goal?
- How does this goal align with my current lifestyle and its features?
- Am I capable of achieving this goal?
- Is this goal currently applicable?

Timely

Goals need a form of due date or a target, this holds us accountable and focused. The main aim of this goal is to ensure that your everyday tasks don't hinder the progress of the goals. Mind Tools (n.d.) suggests answering these questions:

- When is the target?
- How will six months of progress affect the goal?
- What can I achieve in six months from now?
- What do I do today?

What Happens if My Goals Fail?

Don't panic or feel as if the entire process has been a waste, it hasn't. It is okay to fail sometimes; however, failure shouldn't prohibit you from beginning again or scare you into believing that you're too old to properly succeed. Failing and mistakes are natural processes, and everyone goes through them, here are some tips to help you improve:

- Learn from the experience: Taking the time to reflect on what happened before reacting or creating an opinion is extremely important to your overall progress.
- Take a break: This isn't about running away or avoiding the reality of the situation, but by taking a break you're allowing your mind the time to reflect and process what has happened.
- Ask yourself the brutal questions: Don't lie to yourself or disregard facts, we all fail and make mistakes, and the only way to succeed is by

acknowledging why we failed. Most of the time the reason for goals failing is because they are misaligned with what you currently want and need.

- Learn: Now's the time to improve your knowledge and boost your cognitive abilities, failing opens up the mind to a better understanding of what happened and how to improve. Your goal from here on out should be improvement. So, go and learn a new skill or how to improve a current one so that you can succeed the next time.

- Realign your goals: Life gets busy and since our bodies are constantly in the process of changing, it is easy to forget what it is we want when so many other things are happening. Use this opportunity to realign your goals through careful reflection. Journaling can be a great tool for reflection and deeper comprehension.

- Restart: After some time away and before you return to a new schedule, practicing or prioritizing mindfulness is a great place to start to prepare yourself for the next part of the journey.

- Definition: Be clear and firm with yourself about the idea of failure—it doesn't define you and it will never define you. That voice in your head can be tamed with some positivity, there is power in affirmation, and during those moments when you feel you're struggling reach out for support, journal, and practice gratitude.

Chapter 4:
GETTING STARTED: THE BASICS

Regardless of your age, it is extremely important to conduct safety checks whenever you are doing any type of stretching. The great thing about stretching is its relationship to the body and the mind, we know that the mind-body or body-mind—whichever you prefer—connection is a solid foundation. We should all be able to recognize the interconnected relationship between these two factors that are intricately part of us and how they inform one another. According to Hart (n.d., para. 1), it is important to note that "mind is not synonymous with brain. Instead, in our definition, the mind consists of mental states such as thoughts, emotions, beliefs, attitudes, and images. The brain is the hardware that allows us to experience these mental states."

So, when our minds are stressed or fatigued it influences our physical health, specifically our immune system. The same goes for our physical health, injury or illnesses affect our minds, for example, certain physical illnesses can make us more prone to mental health conditions such as depression and anxiety. The aim is to find a balance, and this is why stretching and cultivating flexibility is important, not only are we reducing stress and boosting our serotonin levels but we're also reducing the risk of injury—basically, stretching promotes positive effects in the mind and body without doing double the work. So, it is always recommended to check in with yourself before getting started on the mat.

How to Create a Safe Environment

Let's be realistic, at our age attending classes and specific programs is not always accessible or ideal. Also, it is not financially necessary to splurge. Stretching is a simple process and cost-effective. You honestly don't need much in terms of space and equipment; however, the most important thing you need is a safe space. Now, for some of us cultivating a safe space requires us to move a sofa or a table. Though, this is recommended, daily. So, the first thing to do, before we get stretching is to consider our environment. Also, if you are fortunate enough to have a garden or a garage that's decked out, those are great spaces to practice stretching—since it is out of the way. But if the car needs its spot and the weather cannot accommodate your presence outside, the best thing to do is commit to setting up a space indoors. Note that if you have a garden, you are more than welcome to continue using it when the weather is great.

Home Modifications

When we have cultivated a safe space for stretching, we don't have any reason not to practice—other than health concerns of course. Now, I hate to ask this but when last have you cleared the clutter? Most of the time, the reason why we're so unproductive is due to the environment we are in. If it is cluttered or messy or if that stain wasn't properly cleaned from the rug—regardless of what's happening in your home—it can demotivate you. Also, if the only space you are able to use for your practice sessions is the living room, and it is a little cramped, now is the best time not only to declutter but reconstruct the layout to your benefit. The ultimate goal of the safe space is to feel confident that when you extend an arm or leg you won't hit anything or risk injuring yourself.

Another thing to note is that decluttering is a positive experience, remember that the health of your mind-body connection is contingent on a healthy mindset. If your environment welcomes more negative thoughts than comfort, it may be a sign that it is time to declutter. As previously mentioned, the last thing we want is to constantly move furniture before a session as this can become highly demotivating.

Here are some tips on how to declutter:

- Set realistic goals: Since your goal is to improve your overall health with stretching and achieving flexibility, begin here—with achievable decluttering goals.

- Make a list: This will help you maintain your sanity because decluttering can easily become stressful. So list what needs to go, be moved, or contemplated. For example, you might not want to block the windows and prohibit fresh air from entering the space, so this should be a priority on your list.

- Start small: We've all been there before, the pain of rearranging a room or simply just a sofa can be overwhelming. So, start with something easy, the feeling of accomplishment will energize you to take on the next task.

- Check-in with your emotions: Again, this can be stressful, and it is easy to start feeling sentimental when decluttering. So, make sure to acknowledge these emotions but don't let them distract you from the overall task.

- Set a time: Decluttering tends to run on for hours and days, to maintain your sanity, schedule a specific slot of time to deal with things.

Exercise Accessories

Yoga

When it comes to stretching you don't need to spend a lot on equipment, here are some important tools to have:

Equipment:
- A yoga mat, preferably a sweat-resistant one.
- Yoga blocks and straps to help with stretches.

Attire:
- Anything works but you should opt for comfort and fabric that is stretchable and breathable.
- Footwear:
- Practicing barefoot works, though some people prefer socks.

Tai Chi

Equipment:
- A yoga mat, preferably a sweat-resistant one. However, most people choose to practice outdoors, usually in calm green spaces.
- You don't require any equipment tools for tai chi.

Attire:
- Anything works but opt for comfort and fabric that is stretchable and breathable.

Footwear:

- Practicing barefoot works, though some people prefer socks.

Strength Training

Equipment:

- A yoga mat, preferably a sweat-resistant one.
- Gyms are great because they have most equipment; however, as an older adult and beginner, you don't need much equipment.
- Some light weights are good to have, ankle weights work too.
- You can practice anywhere you are comfortable because your equipment is transportable.

Attire:

- Anything works but opt for comfort and fabric that is stretchable and breathable.
- If you are going to focus on high-intensity workouts (jumps and running), opt for tighter fabrics that won't hinder your movement.

Footwear:

- Comfortable shoes, especially for high-intensity movements.

Trust Your Mind-Body Connection: Be Mindful

You have probably heard the term mindfulness before, a brief search on the internet will display a range of sources on how to be more mindful. Mindfulness is a practice that aims to equip your mental state with awareness of self, and presence, and increase your power of intentionality. At the start of this chapter, we discussed the mind-body connection, and how when the connection is healthy your overall health functions successfully. When starting, mindfulness can feel like a complicated practice, and you might feel as if you are doing it wrong. However, it is the kind of practice that requires constant practice and is a gentle practice that wants to root you in the present.

The Benefits of Mindfulness

Mindfulness has many physical and mental benefits.

- It improves your cognitive abilities, which tend to decrease with age.
- It helps slow down your brain's aging processes, mindfulness requires you to be present and aware of yourself and your surroundings.
- It helps to reduce stress, anxiety, and depression.
- It improves your mood and helps you cultivate a more positive outlook on life.
- It can improve your digestion and blood circulation. This occurs when we practice mindful eating, which allows us to be mindfully aware of the foods, especially their nutritional value, that we consume.
- It can lower your blood pressure.
- It will help you practice acceptance. The truth is that most people—especially women going through menopause—struggle with accepting that their health is not what it was and that it will only continue to decrease. Since mindfulness is about being intentional, it helps us to focus on what truly matters.
- It improves your overall well-being.

How to Practice Mindfulness

There isn't a correct or direct method of practice, ultimately mindfulness is considered a personalized experience between body, mind, and self. There are various sources of information on the internet, especially on YouTube in the form of guided meditations. According to Hoshaw (2022), the easiest technique for mindfulness originates from a 9th-century text from the mystical tradition of Kashmir Shaivism. The text is believed to be written by the sage Vasugupta. However, despite how ancient this technique is, it is still practiced in modern times. It requires the participant to focus on their breath by remaining actively aware of each inhale and exhale. This form of mindfulness is practiced across various forms in life, meaning that you can practice it while you are stuck in traffic or waiting for your appointment in the doctor's office.

When doing your mindfulness practice, it is okay for your mind to wander. This is something you should expect since it happens to everyone. The trick is to acknowledge when your focus is distracted by your thoughts, simply, acknowledge the thought pattern that arose, and mindfully return to your breathing pattern. The overall goal for practicing mindfulness is allowing the practice to recur through various moments in our life, though it is likely that you will begin either seated or lying down comfortably, eventually you'll shift into mindfulness while you are doing the dishes, making the bed, grocery shopping, or going for a walk. The three most significant parts of any mindfulness practice are awareness, distraction, and repetition.

- Awareness: Start becoming more aware of your breath, let it flow through you, and actively observe and feel each inhale and exhale.
- Distraction: Prepare yourself well in advance for distraction, your mind will wander, and it is natural and nothing to beat yourself up about. Only, notice the distraction and then acknowledge it without judgment or comment, and return yourself to your breath. This is key, always return yourself to your breath.

- Repetition: Simply repeat the process, you may want to start with five-minute sessions and progress as you become more comfortable with the process. You could arrange five-minute sessions throughout your day as well.

Mindfulness Activities

Below is a series of activities to incorporate in your life, note that many of these activities are linked to the act of stretching and flexibility.

Breathing Exercises

These are extremely necessary and effective techniques that will help you through any situation at any time. Mindful breathing is equal parts breathing and mindfulness, a great way to practice mindful breathing is during meditation. Meditation enables us to sit, reflect while maintaining gentle awareness of our presence and the environment surrounding us, and breathe. Mindful breathing can calmly help us through difficult situations and experiences; for example, if you are feeling particularly stressed or overwhelmed, the best thing to do is to find a safe space and practice mindful breathing.

A great way to begin is by finding a safe space. Sit or lie down with one hand on your chest and the other on your stomach. Inhale deeply holding your breath for four seconds and then exhale slowly. Be mindful of the sensation of air flowing within you.

Body Scan or Body Awareness

This is another form of mediation that requires you to sit or lie down in a comfortable position—the corpse pose is usually used in this regard—and check in with yourself mentally. Some people often refer to the body scan as a mental X-ray. To perform a body scan, follow the steps below:

- Get cozy and choose the most comfortable position.
- Focus on your breath and close your eyes.
- Choose a spot on your body to begin, top or bottom, if you choose the top of your head, focus on that spot and the sensations related to it while breathing.
- Be aware of those sensations and slowly observe those sensations for about twenty seconds to a minute.
- Acknowledge what you are experiencing, usually, there are emotions associated with these sensations as you continue breathing.
- When you are ready to move on, shift your focus to the next part of your body and repeat the process.
- Now, it is normal for your thoughts to begin drifting, if so, acknowledge them and refocus your mind on your body.

When practicing particular stretches and holding them for a few seconds or a minute, you can follow this same pattern.

Sharpen Your Mind

You are not too old to continue learning or improve your skills. Whether you are interested in learning a new hobby or refining those shabby baking skills, now is the time to see these plans through. This will not only improve your cognitive skills and your brain health but also boost your confidence and levels of joy.

Go for a Walk

Walks are great because they're relaxing as well as a great form of exercise and stretching your limbs. While walking and practicing mindfulness, we're able to observe our surroundings and ourselves within the environment. We're also able to check in with our bodies and notice if there is a particular ache or tenderness. Walking is a great source of exercise and a great form of promoting connection with people.

Don't Forget to Reflect

Journalling is one of the best ways to practice mindfulness. Now, if your excuse is that you have never been much of a writer, it makes no difference since the writing quality doesn't matter. Journalling is not about being the best or descriptive writer, it is about reflecting and checking in on yourself each day. Life is constantly moving, and we forget about ourselves, even in retirement. Reflection is a great tool. It allows us to take a minute and understand what it is we're feeling.

A great way to begin journaling is by writing before bed about your day, it doesn't have to be perfect. The more comfortable you become, the easier the word will flow. You can even start small, and list three things that you were grateful for today.

What makes reflection powerful is its ability to force us to pause; for example, if you find yourself in a stressful situation, the best tip is to walk away. Nobody wants to say anything worth regretting, right? Well, if we're mindful about what is happening during an argument, with enough practice we can stop and reflect on how we're feeling before we respond.

Therapeutic Coloring

The great benefit of coloring again is that you get to spend it with your grandkids—if they are around. However, coloring is intensely therapeutic and allows the mind to focus, through mindfulness, on the act. It will help to reduce stress, improve your focus, and enhance your motor skills.

Connect With Nature

Society is constantly bristling with news and though we care and yearn for its improvement, there is only so much we can do, so take it easy and focus on the environment around you. Your brain health continues to decline, risking a variety of serious mental illnesses. We previously discussed the benefits of taking walks, but you could begin a garden or visit the park and feed the birds. This might be a stereotypical image of old age, but when we can find peace and comfort in routine and our environment, we're not stressing as much.

Daily Positive Affirmations

The idea of affirmations might sound superficial but hear me out, the older we get the more we experience a decrease in compliments. Loneliness is a common trait associated with aging, despite having a partner or family nearby. Our lives are congested with kids and grandkids, and aches. A compliment goes a long way and reading a positive affirmation each day can give you the boost you need. Think of these affirmations as mantras encouraging you each day to better your practice with stretching.

Music Therapy

The trick is to choose calm music, a common stereotype related to music and old age is that we prefer classical music. Now, I'm not going to dispute the authenticity of music—or whatever you prefer to what young folk listen to—but the classical genre procures calmness and emotion. I find that music without strong verbosity is the perfect form to evoke emotion within me. Also, when we find ourselves moved by music, our mind begins to formulate an association between feeling and memory, and this welcomes not only mindfulness but also improves our cognitive abilities.

Guided Sleep Meditation

Sleep complicates with age and we know that sleep is vital to brain health. Guided mediation is led by a teacher either in person or over a device, since it is bedtime, it is likely going to be over your smartphone. Sleep meditation aims to preserve the positivity you acquired—if you followed the previous step that encouraged you to journal before bed and reflect on gratitude—remove all negative thoughts and calm those tense sensations in your body. With constant practice, you will find yourself being able to slip into meditation before bed without the help of an expert.

Understanding Nutrition

Nutrients are chemical compounds found in foods, sourcing the body with sufficient energy to preserve repair and growth throughout its lifetime. Nutrients are complex and are divided into two categories:

- Macronutrients: These are large quantities of nutrients that the body requires to function.
- Micronutrients: These are smaller quantities of nutrients the body needs.

Within these two categories of nutrients are essential nutrients—we use essential to describe them because the body cannot make this nutrient itself and has to source it from foods and supplements—for the body to reach capital function. There are six essential nutrients split between these two categories of nutrients:

- Macronutrients: Carbohydrates, protein, and fat
- Micronutrients: Vitamins and minerals are divided into four categories: water-soluble vitamins, fat-soluble vitamins, microminerals, and trace minerals.

Due to the many changes the body faces with age, a nutritionally dense diet is recommended. A nutritionally dense diet requires the person to mindfully source foods with a higher nutrient count to receive the best value in energy. This nutritionally dense diet must be filled with the finest quality of protein, carbohydrates, fat, vitamins, and minerals. Remember that when nutrition is followed correctly, meaning when we're mindfully strategic about the foods we're eating, we are protecting the body from various illnesses and diseases, while allowing healthy blood circulation, muscle development, bone density, and an operating immune system. Here are ten nutritional changes to improve your diet.

- Eat complex grains: These are carbohydrates, and the trick is to switch refined bread and pasta for more filling grains.
  - Choose foods like quinoa, amaranth, buckwheat, oats, etc.
- Eat more fish: This is a great source of protein and healthy fats like omega-3 and can help reduce inflammation.
  - Aim to eat fish two to three times a week.
- Monitor your sodium levels: The higher the intake of sodium the higher the risk of heart disease, so be mindful of the salt you are adding.
  - A good tip is to stop using the saltshaker and opt for fresh herbs to build flavor and balance.
- Enjoy foods with higher protein levels: This is going to aid your muscle mass development.
  - Choose foods like steak, fish, chicken, turkey, tofu, lentils, quinoa, etc.
- Cook your meals: This is a great way to practice mindfulness about the food you are consuming and can help you avoid extra sugars, salts, and oils.
- Choose high-calcium foods: This is to improve your bone density by serving as a preventive measure against osteoporosis and help prevent fracture and injury.
  - A Mediterranean diet is often chosen because it is comprised of cheese, grains, veggies, fish, etc. while reducing the processed food content.

- Stop drinking soda: You don't need soda or sugary drinks, switch to lighter and more nutritional options, and make sure you are getting enough water.
- Eat the rainbow: It may seem superficial, but aiming for a colorful plate of food will keep you in check to source the nutritional ones.
    - Always add fruits and veggies, sweet potatoes, greens, beets, eggplants, etc.
- Eat only when you are hungry: To do this we must be mindful of the foods we're eating.
- Choose whole foods: Not only will this nourish your body and help your metabolism, but if you are consuming the right foods, you will be fueled and energized throughout the day.

A Note on Resilience

Resilience is about bouncing back from challenges and difficulties, not necessarily quickly, but rather infused with the same determined abilities of before. I've been thinking about resilience and how much we need it during these moments in our lives. Stretching in some way is about maintaining resilience throughout each moment and particularly during the inability of the movement. Remember that resilience is about sourcing ways to adapt to the situation, your first impression of hardship or failure shouldn't be giving up. Instead, always take your time, we discussed this in the previous chapter, and reflect. Not only will this form of resilience affect your health, but it is going to positively affect your mental health, which in return will lower those levels of depression and anxiety. You will feel a boost in your overall mood and your self-esteem will increase, affecting your confidence.

Always remember to stay connected to those around you, especially where your support systems are and if you are struggling to openly communicate, find a counselor or therapist to discuss your emotions. Remember resilience isn't focused on avoiding or disregarding, be honest with yourself about what you are going through. Another important factor about sustaining resilience is that you must prioritize yourself and self-care. Make sure that your diet and fitness regime are on track and that you are cultivating the time for sleep, specifically rest. Also, let's be clear rest is not the equivalent of sleep. So, be generous with yourself.

We want to thank you for purchasing this book. If you have found it helpful, please go to Amazon and write a brief review. This would be so appreciated and will give other seniors an idea of what this book is all about.

And please be looking for other books for seniors that we will be publishing in the very near future.

Seniors are our primary focus, and your input will be most appreciated.

Nick and Nora

Chapter 5:
FLEXIBILITY EXERCISES FOR SENIORS

The main reason we want to strengthen our flexibility is that it prohibits the risk of falling and the fall-related injuries that we, as seniors, are more susceptible to. However, people often dismiss the importance of flexibility since they see it as merely a way of bending or folding, instead of a practice that also focuses on patience and breathing. In order to become flexible, we must commit to serious stretching, which means understanding the importance of stretching and treating it as part of our commitment to bettering our overall health.

Stretching Essentials

Here are a few things to keep in mind before beginning your stretching routine, remember that incorrect stretching will hinder and put you at a risk for injury.

- Strive for symmetry: We are all different and regardless of the progress we make, our flexibility won't match. Also, it is completely natural to feel as if one side of your body is more flexible than the other side, balancing them out will take time.

- Focus on major muscle groups: Take your time and be mindful of your movements, aim for stretches that incorporate various muscles. However, don't rush and practice each movement before progressing to the next step.

- Don't bounce: Stretching is a fluid movement, for example, yoga uses breath to help you move into the next movement. So, avoid any static "bouncing" movements.

- Hold your stretch: Remember to breathe mindfully throughout each step and hold each of the stretches for about thirty seconds; if, however, this is too long, start with twenty seconds and work your way up.

- Don't aim for pain: If it hurts, stop immediately. You shouldn't feel any pain while you are stretching but some tightness after the stretch when you first begin is normal.

- Make your stretch sport specific: If you are performing a particular workout session; for example, doing a strength upper body workout, try some dynamic stretching for those specific muscle groups.

- Stay committed: It is a process that will require patience, though rest is fine and understandable, don't take long breaks in between sessions, you'll only sabotage your progress and risk losing all the benefits you have acquired. Remember that progress is permanent, you must consistently work to maintain it.

What Are The Best Warm-Up And Stretching Strategies?

Keep in mind that each of us is different and the warm-up routine you prefer will be individual and based on the workout you are going to practice. Remember that a warm-up is there to prepare your body for the workout, it warms up your body temperature as well as your heart, muscles, and joints.

Is Stretching the Equivalent of A Warm-Up?

An important difference between warming up and stretching is that the former involves a series of activities to increase your heart rate and get your blood pumping, whereas the latter focuses on holding a specific stretch. However, we know that stretching is split into four different forms, each with its own warmup routine. It is important to always warm up before you stretch, even yoga includes warm-up stretches to get you into the most flexible stretches. Dynamic stretching is a great form of stretching, an example of productive dynamic stretching happens when you are activating your glutes before an intense lower body workout. Be practical when it comes to stretches, if you are going to be holding static poses for a while, warm up those joints before practicing those stretches.

What Are the Benefits of Warming Up?

Beyond getting your heart rate up, warming up has the following benefits:

- It helps to increase your flexibility.
- It lowers your risk of injury.
- It increases your blood flow and oxygen levels.

- It helps improve your performance and positively impacts your exercises.
- It helps improve your range of motion.
- It helps to reduce the risk of pain and tension.

How Long Should A Warmup Be?

A warm-up session shouldn't be too long or too short, varying between five to fifteen minutes depending on how tight your muscles are and what you are preparing your body for. However, your warm-up should never run as long as your actual workout.

What Are Good Upper Body Warm-Up Exercises?

The best exercises are the ones that incorporate minimal movement and activate a series of muscles, upper body warm-up exercises are best used when doing strength training. The five movements listed below are great exercises to practice before beginning an upper body workout, they not only activate the right muscle groups but are also used to strengthen your balance. Remember that a good warm-up for the upper body isn't reliant on using weights; it focuses on using your body weight to create tension or resistance bands. According to McCoy, "A solid upper-body warm-up also increases your range of motion and thus allows you to perform movements in your workout to their full extent. This, in turn, boosts the strengthening benefits of your workout" (2021, para.1).

Remember that the upper-body warm-up aims to increase your heart rate while activating your core and muscles. When our core and muscles are activated, it benefits and strengthens the spine, this is great because our body is reliant on our legs, and therefore our spine, to get by throughout the day. This slightly neglects the core and our lower back. "After all, you need a strong core to help you perform upper-body exercises like the overhead press and the row since your core muscles help keep you stable and transfer power to heft that weight" (McCoy, 2021, para.1).

Upper Body Warm-Up Exercises

The pull-apart

The pull-apart uses a resistant band and it helps warm up your upper back and rotator cuff muscles—these are muscles and joints located around your shoulders. This exercise benefits the body by preparing your chest and shoulders and working on your stability. Here's how to begin:

- Stand tall with a slight bend in your knees to protect your joints, with your legs hip-width apart, and holding the resistance band in both hands.
- Raise both hands with your arms straight, keep a slight bend in the elbows, face your palms downward, and keep your arms about five to six inches apart.
- The band should have slight resistance, begin pulling the band apart. Widen your arms as far as they can, the aim is to create a T position with your arms expanded.
- Once you have the T position, hold the stretch for about two seconds and slowly return your arms to the center. This counts as 1 rep.
- Do six to ten reps.

Incline push-up

This warm-up activates your pectoral muscles, some parts of your lower chest, and also your core. This variation is an easier version of a push-up. You'll be performing the pushup at an incline angle, meaning that you can use the wall, a table, a chair, or a stable box. The higher your chest is the easier the exercise. Here's how to perform this exercise:

- Decide what your incline is going to be, a stable box, the wall, a step, or even a countertop.
- Start in a high plank, so your hands are flat and shoulder-width apart. Remember to check your form, your shoulders should be hovering directly over your wrists.
- Spread your legs hip-width apart behind you. Be mindful of your muscles, especially your core and glutes.
- Bend from your elbows and try to get your chest close to the wall—or whatever you are using.
- Do six to ten reps.

Chest opener or thread the needle

This is also a yoga stretch and is considered a great shoulder opener, it releases tension in the shoulders, neck, and upper back. This positive effect increases your range of motion. Here's how to practice this exercise:

- Start in a tabletop position, be mindful of your form; stack your shoulders over your wrists and your hips over your knees.
- Lift your right arm upwards, naturally opening up the side of your body, you'll feel a stretch running through your side. Take the arm back, as if

returning it to the tabletop position; however, twist and move the arm underneath your chest.

- As your right arm continues stretching inward, bend your left arm to allow this stretch.
- Do five reps before switching sides.

Squat thrust

The squat thrust movement is a modification of the burpee. This is a great warm-up exercise because it activates multiple parts of the body and ultimately provides you with some cardio which boosts your heart rate. However, there are many parts to the exercise, so be mindful of your form throughout. It is best to start slow until you are comfortable with each section. Here's how to perform the squat thrust:

- Stand with your feet hip-width apart, your core engaged, and your hands at your sides.
- Squat down and place your hands on the floor, they should be shoulder width apart and firm, then jump or step back into a high plank position.
- Jump or step back toward your hands, finding your squat position and as you rise, lift your arms into the air. This is one rep.
- Do six to ten reps.

Tabletop plank

This is a modification of the plank, though some may argue that it is more intense. This movement will activate your core, spine, shoulders, and muscles. Here's how to perform it:

- Find a tabletop position, make sure that your shoulders are hovering over your wrists and your hips over your knees.
- Press your hands firmly into the ground as you begin to lift your toes, tucking them in. Hover your knees and body inches above the ground.
- Your back should be flat and weight evenly distributed.
- Hold for ten to twenty-five seconds.

Why Should I Focus on My Form?

The most important thing to understand about your form when stretching or doing any form of movement is that poor form puts you at risk of injury. No exercise should be rushed, you should always start at the beginner's level before proceeding to the next level and remember to always warm up before and after any workout. Time and patience are essential skills to have when beginning any new activity. Having good form will -

- contribute toward a safer overall workout.
- make your workout feel a lot easier.
- help you improve your breathing techniques.
- make sure you target the correct muscles.
- reduce the risk of injury.

Common FAQ's About Flexibility

I've tried improving my flexibility before, but it has never worked out for me. I'm older now, will it work now and what difference will it make?

For starters, flexibility is an eventual achievement that varies in range. This means that though you may reach certain levels of flexibility it is possible never to reach the same level of flexibility as others. Our level of flexibility and range of motion differ from person to person.

Now, when it comes to stretching, we are aiming to increase our range of motion, which ultimately requires time and motivation. There are various reasons stretching may have failed for you in the past, but anyone can succeed with the correct practice and honest levels of motivation.

Stretching offers the aging body a variety of benefits, and one of the goals is to reduce the risk of falling due to our decline in balance.

If I hold my stretches for longer periods, it will advance my range of flexibility?

Not exactly, though the goal is to hold the pose for an extended timeframe. This shouldn't be forced, and you should aim to hold the pose for about twenty seconds and work your way toward longer periods.

Do I have to stretch every day in order to reap the benefits of flexibility?

No, the benefits of stretching aren't necessarily allocated with each day of practice. Also, if you are going to practice every day you run the risk of severe injury which will prohibit you from continuing your process. Another thing to remember is that stretching overused muscles won't improve their range of motion.

I don't need to warm up before stretching, because it is the same thing, right?

This can be tricky to fully understand, and ultimately depends on the type of stretching you are doing. A noted difference between stretching and warming up is that the former encourages a range of motion and extension toward flexibility. Whereas the latter aims to prepare the body for a workout routine by increasing the heart rate, blood supply, and oxygen to working muscles.

What's the best way to incorporate flexibility into my life now?

There isn't an exact correct way to introduce stretching to your life, if you feel that now's the time, then I encourage you to begin. However, it is best to choose a specific time of day, including stretching in your daily schedule makes you accountable to see it through while also creating a new habit. A great time to start is at the beginning of the day. However, note that if you are practicing other fitness routines, allow stretching before and after your workout.

Should I stretch an injured muscle?

This is tricky and entirely dependent on the severity of your injury. The first thing to do is determine how severe the injury is, and if it needs medical assistance, visit your general practitioner. If you don't feel you need a medical practitioner, observe the sensations that occur when you begin stretching, if the injury hurts, stop stretching that muscle. A sore muscle usually requires two to four days of rest, you can also apply the PRICE method—Protection, Rest, Ice, Compression, and Elevation. Now, if the injury continues to be a problem, visit your practitioner if you haven't already.

What is the stretch reflex?

The stretch reflex, or the myotatic reflex, refers to the contraction of muscles when we're practicing passive stretching. So, when the stretch is activated the muscle—, the inside of the muscle—will stretch as well. This happens to prevent any form of injury, when the stretch is activated, a message is sent to the spinal cord. This message informs the relevant parties of the muscle lengthening and adapts the rest of the body to the stretch, improving the range of flexibility.

Is there a thing such as overstretching?

Yes, there is. We previously discussed whether it is beneficial to practice stretching daily and noted that this is dependent on your body and how long you have been practicing stretching. However, to prevent overstretching you must incorporate a mindful pace, checking in with yourself and your body to understand if it is tender or tight in certain places. Don't rush the process, take it slow.

How important is the correct breathing techniques for flexibility training?

Breathing is key to our ultimate success, breathing and stretching are significantly paired— in the next chapter, we will discuss the benefits of yogic breathing. Breathing is tied to the practice of mindfulness, and it helps us monitor ourselves throughout each stretch.

Should I follow a particular diet alongside my flexibility routine?

An overall nutritional diet will work best for you. Remember that the decline in your health ultimately forces you to make better life choices, especially dietary choices. So, take the time to be mindful of the food you are consuming.

Chapter 6:
YOGA

Yoga continues to rise in popularity. Especially since the media presents society as stricken with constant mindless movement, for which the cure is overall prioritizing our health through a series of self-care practices that aim to preserve particular pillars of health. Self-care is defined as an essential skill that each of us should acquire to influence success within our lifestyle. Self-care pillars are often categorized into multiple parts; however, these differ from person to person. This is due to each of us requiring various needs or necessities to cultivate a healthy lifestyle. Yoga usually falls into the self-care pillar focused on fitness. The great thing about yoga is that it is closely associated with mindfulness.

Yoga is an ancient practice that can be traced back 5000 years to Northern India and endured a series of refinement principles to its craft since then. Modern yoga is known or treated as a complementary health approach to maintaining health. There are over 100 styles of yoga practices, these include:

- Hatha yoga
- Aerial yoga
- Hot Yoga
- Iyengar yoga
- Restorative yoga

- Yin yoga
- Ashtanga vinyasa yoga
- Chair yoga
- Prenatal yoga

However, these are just a few yoga styles practiced across the world. A benefit often associated with yoga is its ability to delay the body's response to aging. Many yoga practitioners will declare that though their range of motion and flexibility has increased, practicing yoga is not about delaying aging. If anything, it is about slowing down the inevitable.

The Benefits of Practicing Yoga

There are various benefits to practicing yoga, particularly as a senior.

- Your flexibility will improve with practice.
- It serves as a great tool for stress relief, and this will improve your mental health.
- Your physical strength will improve. Yoga relies on a series of plank movements, and these are great exercises to enhance your upper body and core strength.
- Your quality of life will improve, this means that when your emotions, mental health, and physical health are in balance your overall well-being flourishes.
- Your balance will improve, and this will reduce your risk of falling.
- Your sleep will improve, and this will in turn positively affect your brain health.
- Yoga will boost your mood and improve your self-esteem.
- You will develop better posture and body awareness.

- It will positively affect your heart health and reduce your blood pressure, cholesterol, and blood sugar levels.
- It will improve your body image.

How Does One Go About Beginning A Yoga Journey?

Even though yoga can be practiced at home and many other people swear by the financial benefits of simply following along to a practice on YouTube, it is recommended that seniors seek professional in-person help, especially those who are new to the practice. **Questions About Yoga**

What exactly is yoga?

The simplest way to understand yoga is by considering it a system that is built to promote balance in the body and mind. There are two important aspects to yoga (the system), one is focused on postures which are called asanas, and the other is focused on breathing exercises called pranayama—we'll get into both the asanas and pranayama techniques in a bit. When these two aspects of yoga are successfully enacted, yoga can be used in practices like mindfulness, self-awareness, and reflection.

As a beginner which style should I start with?

One great aspect of yoga is that there are over a hundred yoga styles, and you can decide which style works for you. So, you'll likely need to engage in some trial and error before settling on your chosen style. However, when you sign up for a class, it is best to enquire which style of yoga is being practiced. Again, research is key to your success. However, beginner yoga will ease you into the practice and introduce you to a variety of styles. Once you advance to the beginner stage of your journey, you'll be able to decide which flow or which variety of flows are better suited for you.

How do I know if I'm doing it right?

This is why attending a class is important. I know that we previously discussed the benefits of constructing a home-based workout space; however, the most important thing about becoming more agile and fit is form. Without proper form, you are setting yourself up for failure and severe injury. So, it is best to first sign up for a beginner class and learn. Once you have learned properly and trust yourself, you can continue this practice at home.

With the help of an instructor, you can learn proper alignment and techniques to improve alignment. Remember that through mindfulness, we are aiming to construct body awareness, which takes time and trust and shouldn't be rushed. So, don't be too hard on yourself if you can't do everything perfectly on the first try.

It is also important to remember that yoga shouldn't hurt, so if you find yourself in a particular pose and it hurts or there are shooting pains, inform your instructor. Another benefit to attending a beginner program is that it will allow you to ask questions, so I encourage you to always ask.

How often should I practice yoga?

During the beginning phase of your practice, once a week is perfectly fine. You can then build up to two to three times a week, which is the perfect number of practice sessions. Some people who have been practicing yoga for years, even enjoy practicing it each day. In terms of how long a session should be; though yoga is about a fluid motion of movement through various poses (asanas), it can range between 10 to 40-minute sessions. Even though stretching every day isn't necessarily bad, incorrectly practicing a thirty to forty-minute session every day can have severe effects on your body.

However, if you practiced thirty to forty-minute sessions two times a week, you could include light stretching which takes up about five to ten minutes each. The focus shouldn't be on duration but simply managing to build consistency through positive movement.

When is the best time of day to practice yoga?

This is dependent on your schedule, some people prefer stretching as soon as they wake up, while others prefer a light practice before bed. So, this is your decision; however, some forms of activity are known to boost and energize us, so if practice before bed prohibits sleep it might be best to practice yoga in the morning.

Should I eat before or after yoga?

Again, this may vary from person to person but to be safe, it is best to stop eating at least two hours before you begin practicing yoga. Water and light beverages are fine to consume, but due to the twists and movements of the postures, your digestion may suffer.

Can I still practice yoga even if I have a health condition?

Yes, but first have a chat with your medical practitioner. Yoga is safe and people with various medical illnesses are known to practice it successfully, but it is best to check first.

Are there any side effects I should know about?

Well, when yoga is practiced correctly there shouldn't be any side-effects. Now, even when practiced correctly, a few weeks after you start your body will change and there will be some momentary stiffness or aches—as occurs with most fitness routines. However, these shouldn't be viewed as side effects. If during practice you feel soreness, inform your instructor.

How flexible do I have to be to practice yoga?

No, it is okay if you can't touch your toes. Yoga will improve your flexibility.

Will yoga allow me to lose weight?

Yoga can help with weight loss but also with weight maintenance. However, though certain styles of yoga are faster-paced, yoga is not the most effective tool for weight loss. When breath and body are successfully paired, detoxification can occur within your digestive tract, and your stress and anxiety levels will also decrease. When you are in a healthier mindset, your body is more perceptible to functionality.

Additional Tips to Keep in Mind About A Yoga Class

The world is filled with yoga classes. Research is extremely important, something to look out for is yoga aimed at seniors. If there's no precise wording associated with yoga for seniors, you could chat with the administrator at the class or the instructor about whether or not the class is suited for you. Gentle yoga classes are also a good place to start, though they aren't specifically aimed at beginners, these classes focus on slower movements. Other styles of yoga worth trying are chair yoga, restorative yoga, or Hatha yoga—all of these are focused on slower and more controlled movement. Don't be discouraged if one specific style doesn't seem to work out for you. Also, talk to your instructor about any health complications that you are currently facing; for example, if you are recovering from the aftereffects of an infection that is affecting your breathing or recently had an injury or fall. Due to these complications, certain postures may be impossible to practice. Also, because there are a variety of postures, informing your instructor about your struggles with arthritis or vertigo will help them determine which alternative posture is best suited for your health. The same goes for muscle stiffness or soreness, always inform your instructor.

Another tip is to know your limits with practice or rather what the preventive abilities of yoga are. Many people hear, through reports carelessly spread through the media or society, that there are various ways to reduce the effects of aging—we call this anti-aging. However, yoga, and any form of exercise really, cannot prohibit aging. Its only goal is to promote effective strategies to delay the harsh effects of aging—basically, you're still going to age, just bit slower. Yoga is just one step, remember that age affects your muscles and tendons. Yoga cannot restore this damage; you would need to introduce strength-based training to your daily routine. Remember that yoga will challenge your body; however, it doesn't possess enough quality or sustenance to create muscle development. Your tendons are also known to suffer great loss, though yoga will increase your range of flexibility it cannot however repair tendon damage. A decline in balance is normal with aging and if your agility is still on the mend, it is best to begin with chair yoga or yoga that allows you to use the wall.

The same goes for people suffering from osteoporosis, certain poses that are reliant on the rounding of the back, such as the cat-cow pose, or the forward fold should be avoided. Engaging in these poses can cause severe injuries that can be harmful to your health and set your progress back. It may be slightly discouraging watching other people progress easily but remember that each of us has a different body and levels of health. The truth is that aging is a stressful experience and readapting can be difficult and sometimes, off-putting, you might even question whether or not it is worth it to pursue optimal health at this age. We're often warned that when we start aging, we will endure intense loneliness despite the presence of loved ones around us and that the possibility of depression also increases. However, this is where the mind-body connection comes in; by practicing yoga, you can also improve your mental health.

The impact of these challenges on the body can be overwhelming, this is why attending a yoga class can be extremely beneficial. It opens up our experience without the pressure of actually making friends or conversation. But during these yoga classes, we're surrounded by people who are experiencing the same complications we are. And though you don't have to make friends, you will gradually realize that aging just opens you up to a new community.

Breathing Techniques: Yogic Breathing

Yogic breathing is also referred to as pranayama and it is described as the practice of controlling the breath. This is an ancient breathing technique that originated in India and is used in yoga and meditation as a way to help participants focus on the mind. Yogic breathing techniques can also be used for mindfulness, progressive muscle relaxation, mindfulness-based stress reduction (MBSR), body scan meditations, and breathwork classes.

Benefits of Yogic Breathing

In addition to aiding in yoga practice, yogic breathing has many other benefits.

Nervous System Regulation

By practicing yogic breathing, we are activating the parasympathetic system or our automatic nervous systems. This state is also known as the rest and digest state. The automatic nervous system is comprised of nerves that are in charge of our automatic physical responses and functions, like breathing, digesting, and heart rate. This is where yogic breathing improves the function of our nervous system:

- The vagus nerve is the physical response to the physical environment. The vagus nerve takes up 75% of our automatic nervous system and also helps the body relax. Paired with yogic breathing, for example, humming breath stimulates the vagus nerve and helps your body and mind find a space of calmness.

- The amygdala is the part of the brain that controls your emotions and emotional responses, when our emotions are flustered it triggers an anxious or fearful response in the amygdala, when paired successfully with yogic breathing we're able to focus on our breath and reduce the emotional activity occurring.
- The locus coeruleus is in charge of producing a hormone known as norepinephrine that helps regulate the nervous system; yogic breathing can help restore these levels with focus.

Cardiovascular Function

When yogic breathing is slowed down it can have a positive effect on the cardiovascular system. Now, our automatic systems (mentioned above) manage the cardiovascular system. So, when yogic breathing triggers the vagus nerve it relaxes the automatic nervous system, and this helps manage cardiac functions. Here are some cardiovascular benefits:

- It lowers your heart rate.
- It lowers your blood pressure.
- It will increase your heart rate.
- It will increase oxygen levels in the blood.

Respiratory Function

By slowing down and focusing on your breath, you are ultimately improving your respiratory functions. Yogic breathing will increase your lung capacity, its strength, and relax the muscles. Also, when you engage the diaphragm through yogic breathing, it strengthens your pelvic floor muscles, stabilizes your core muscles, and helps your ribs and spine which will reduce lower back pain.

Mental Health

Yogic breathing will improve your stress and anxiety levels by reducing your dependency on launching into a flight or fight response.

Emotional Regulation

Emotional regulation refers to our management and response to our emotions. When practicing yogic breathing, because you are focused on the present moment, you will notice that your emotions begin to arise. The easiest option is to ignore the emotions we don't want to deal with, but when we're practicing mindfulness, we know that these emotions will constantly arise and all we have to do is acknowledge them. Yogic breathing is a great source for managing these emotions and will help us eventually accept those emotions.

Types of Yogic Breathing

There are nine types of yogic breathing, some are used to clear the mind and preserve meditation practices while others are known to build up energy. All nine types of yogic breathing rely on three interrelated parts: inhalation, retention, and exhalation. The only difference is that each of these nine types of yogic breathing requires a different technique and incorporates those types of breathing differently. Differences between these nine types include the depth of your inhalation, the length of retention, and the force of the exhale. Now, if you have an instructor, it is likely that they will help ease you through these various breathing techniques. Don't forget to ask questions and to understand why certain breathing techniques are strategically employed with certain styles of yoga. Below we'll look into Dirga Pranayama's, or three-part, breathing technique.

Three-Part Breath (Dirga Pranayama)

This technique is aimed at relaxing and calming the mind and is often incorporated into meditation or more gentle practices of yoga. *Dirga* refers to the feeling of completeness or fullness because this type of breathing allows you to use your lungs to their full capacity. This is considered to be one of the more popular types of breathing.

There are three parts to this technique:

- The first part requires you to safely prepare your environment, remove all distractions, and find a comfortable spot. Whether you are seated or lying down, close your eyes and begin to observe your breathing. The aim is to observe first and not impact this natural breathing pace.
    - After a minute, begin to deepen your breath, inhale, and exhale through your nose.
    - On the inhale fill your stomach with breath and upon exhale empty it completely.
    - Tip: Pull your belly button toward your spine on the exhale to make sure you are releasing all that air.
    - Repeat this for five breaths.
- The second part requires you to deepen your inhales and repeat the process as before; however, when you reach the point of fullness, breathe in a little more. The aim is to feel the rib cage expand and separate.
    - Exhale by releasing all the air from your rib cage first, feeling those bones suction back together as your belly button pulls in toward your spine.
    - Repeat this for five breaths.

- The third part requires you to not only the belly and ribs but also your heart.
  - Begin to inhale, breathing in to inflate the rib cage, and then breathe in a little more to expand your chest and feel it rise. You want your heart to be full of air.
  - When you begin to exhale, release the air from your heart, ribs, and then belly with the belly button pulling in toward the spine.
  - Practice this process at your own pace and continue toward finding comfortability.
  - Repeat ten times.

How to Practice Yogic Breathing

Yogic breathing can be practiced anywhere and at any time. Besides the simplest approach of just sitting or lying down, you can practice your breathing with significant yoga poses.

Yoga Poses

Side Warrior Pose

- Stand sideways on your mat and step out to the side with your left foot (about four to five feet).
- Turn your left foot out toward ninety degrees—ideally, your foot should be facing the top side of your mat,
- Turn your body toward the same direction and begin to lower yourself to the point of comfort.
- The left leg will begin to bend. Remember to incorporate your breath with this movement and if you can lift both arms straight into the sky.

- Keep your right leg extended behind you with a slight bend in the knee.

Reclining twist

- Begin by lying on your back with your legs extended and one hand placed on your heart and the other on your belly.
- Take a minute and focus on your breathing.
- Extend your arms out to the side, with your palms facing up, inhale, and pull your knees into your chest.
- Lift them to a tabletop position with your knees bent and gently lower them to the right side before returning them to the center and over to the other side.
- Base each movement on an inhale and exhale.

Gate Pose

- On your knees and facing forward, extend your left leg out to the side.
- Lengthen the muscle and balance the leg on its heel with the toes pointing upwards.
- Check your alignment, especially your hips.

Flowing Mountain pose

- Stand up straight with your legs pressed together.
- Inhale, and raise your arms with your head and vision facing upwards toward the sky or ceiling.
- With an exhale lower your arms at a ninety-degree angle.
- On your next inhale lift the arms and repeat the motion.

Chapter 7:
TAI CHI: THE ART OF MOVEMENT

Tai chi is a low-impact form of exercise that focuses on deepening your breath while doing a series of gentle motions. Tai chi is often referred to as 'meditation in motion' due to the ability breathing has to sustain energy. It is an ancient practice that is centuries old and rooted in traditional Chinese medicine. You have probably seen images of people practicing tai chi and repeating phrases about being one with the wind or like water. An interesting fact about tai chi is that it was originally designed as a self-defense practice and a tool to promote inward clarity and peace. This is quite fitting in our quest to introduce tai chi to combat balance disorders. Tai chi continues to be an important pillar of traditional Chinese medicine and focuses on balancing your body's energy and using this energy restoratively and productively. The energy used in tai chi is referred to as qi and when your qi (energy) is balanced your body is in optimal function.

The Benefits of Tai Chi

Practicing tai chi can provide a wide range of benefits.

Reducing Stress Levels

A study focused on 'healthy but stressed people ' investigated tai chi's influence on these people's lives for twelve weeks and found that their anxiety levels decreased significantly more than other forms of practice (Cleveland Clinic, 2022). Mindfulness is another component used when practicing tai chi, due to the gentle composure required by each movement.

Improving Balance

A review of studies focused on tai chi and balance found that those who regularly practiced tai chi had fifty percent fewer falls than those who didn't engage in the practice (Cleveland Clinic, 2022).

Supporting Brain Health

Brain health is extremely important, especially since the older we get the more our brains experience a reduction in function. A study focused on people in their sixties found that those who practiced tai chi daily for 12 weeks were able to more smoothly switch between tasks than those without the practice (Cleveland Clinic, 2022). The study also found that the prefrontal cortex—the region of the brain responsible for critical thinking and decision-making skills—had more activity. Tai chi is known to significantly improve memory in older adults when practiced regularly for three times a week.

Supporting Mental Health

A study interested in older adults with depression closely observed the effect of anti-depressants paired with tai chi and found that symptoms decreased (Cleveland Clinic, 2022).

Dealing With Fibromyalgia Pain

Fibromyalgia is a chronic disease that causes one to endure severe pain throughout the body. A randomized study observed the effects of tai chi compared to aerobic exercise on people suffering from fibromyalgia and found that tai chi produced incredible results, offering relief to patients (Cleveland Clinic, 2022).

Helping With Knee Osteoarthritis

Weekly tai chi practice can aid pain related to osteoarthritis in the knees. The Arthritis Foundation and the American College of Rheumatology (ACR) recommend tai chi as a beneficial tool for managing and reducing pain (Cleveland Clinic, 2022).

Other Benefits

Other benefits include:

- It is affordable, you don't need equipment or an expensive class. There are numerous videos online to get you started.
- It is a low-impact workout, so it is not too strenuous, and though it doesn't offer the same levels of flexibility as yoga, it is a great filler exercise to use on active rest days.
- It is highly accessible, so there's no reason why you shouldn't be able to practice it.

What Are The Five Types of Tai Chi?

Tai chi is divided into five primary forms or styles, and though each one follows the same system and is guided by the same premise, they have slight variations in style.

Chen

The Chin style of tai chi was developed in the 1600s. It is considered to be the oldest style of tai chi which ultimately makes it the original style and was created by the Chen family who lived in the Chen Village (Gould, 2021). It "is characterized by a combination of slow and then quick movements, including jumping, kicking, and striking. Chen also utilizes a movement called "silk reeling," which is essentially a spiral-esque, flowing movement" (Gould, 2021, para.3). The silk reeling movement serves as the foundation for the Chen-style tai chi.

Yang

Yang is regarded as the most popular style of tai chi and is the most practiced style of tai chi. It originated in the 1800s, was based on the Chen style, and is named after its founder Yang Lu-Ch'an (Gould, 2021). The key difference between the two styles is that this one focuses on improving flexibility through grand sweeping movements that its often displayed with graceful motion. The Chen style is quicker paced and because the Yang is about slow and controlled movement it is more accessible for all ages and fitness levels.

Wu

This style of tai chi was created by Wu Ch'uan-yu who had originally trained under the Yang style. Wu is considered to be a popular style and mostly focuses on practicing extension movements that allow the body to either lean forward or backward as opposed to remaining centered in one position. This style improves balance significantly.

Sun

Sun Lutang developed this style of tai chi; they were Confucian and Taoist scholars who bore incredible expertise in different forms of Chinese martial arts. This version, probably due to Sun's background in martial arts, requires more footwork compared to the other movements. Watching this style of tai chi performed resembles a choreographed dance.

Hao

This style of tai chi is considered to be the least popular, mainly due to the level of control and skill needed to accomplish it. Due to its complicated nature, it is not recommended for beginners, and it is best to first ease through the other four styles before trying this style (Gould, 2022).

What Is The Aim of Tai Chi?

Tai chi aims to reinvigorate your relationship with the environment. We have already learned that the environment we find ourselves in is one of the major contributors to stress. The reality for most of us is that we can't just pick up and leave, not everyone is this fortunate, and you may just be choosing to avoid your situation. Self-awareness is essential and tai chi is a great practice to help re-establish it in our lives, especially when the environment we're in is stressful. Ultimately, tai chi aims to make you one with nature again. If we're mindfully connected to our environment, it means that the usual stressors won't hinder us as much. Tai chi not only teaches us how to observe before reacting but also how to slow down our fast-paced life. Below, the principles of tai chi have been divided into three main sections.

Movement Control

Tai chi is focused on gentle movements that are strategically slowed down to help you connect your body and mind. It aims to create the sensation of serenity which strengthens your inner energy.

The key is to move as if you are moving against resistance and let each movement infuse you with inner power and peace.

Body Structure

T a strong posture that stabilizes the muscles as it supports the spine. Good posture opens up your internal body and allows expansion between your organs, helping you feel stronger and boosting your mood. Your cultivated energy (qi) will flow better if your body is aligned and without tension.

Be mindful as you transfer weight between each movement. Balance is an essential concept of tai chi.

Internal Components

Tai chi can help you develop a sense of calmness and inner peace. You can also use mindfulness to observe and reflect on how each movement makes you feel. Your energy (qi) finds great effect within you, the more balanced your body is—in terms of functionality and health—the more powerful your energy becomes. Lam (n.d.) states that despite the simplicity of these principles when tai chi is practiced with intentionality and purpose it releases profound effects.

Chapter 8:
STRENGTH TRAINING: A PILLAR OF STABILITY

⸻◇◇◇⸻

It doesn't matter if you have never lifted a weight or committed to an intense cardio-based workout before. If you are entirely new to the practice of exercise that's even better. Consider strength training for seniors as a challenge, a skill you want to equip yourself with, and a goal you want to accomplish. According to Sportsspt, due to the decline in health, our muscles begin to shrink and lose mass, which causes a loss of elasticity and slows down recovery from exercise. "Strength training can help seniors counteract the natural effects aging has on muscles. Research shows that strength training can even help to reverse some symptoms of chronic diseases like sarcopenia and osteoporosis" (Sportsspt, 2020. para.1). So, if your workout doesn't include strength training, you are missing out on vital benefits. Strength training not only helps to slow down age-related muscle loss, but it increases our range in mobility and manages good bone health. Also, those who include strength training in their workout routine will notice improvements in balance, falls, risk, and mental health.

Here are the benefits of strength training for seniors:

- It helps reduce symptoms of age-related diseases: Research has indicated that once we reach forty significant losses in muscle loss has already begun (Sportsspt, 2020).

- It strengthens your bones: Strength training develops your muscle mass while adding weight to your body.
- Your core muscles will strengthen, reducing your joint pain.
- Your overall mental well-being will improve.

Is Strength Training Safe for Seniors?

Believe me, I get your concern, strength training from the perspective of an older adult can seem untrustworthy and frightening. But strength training is safe, as long as you do your part, remembering to check in with yourself and your form throughout the exercise. Research, which was inclusive of seniors who suffered from disease and illness, has confirmed the safety of strength training for seniors (Sportsspt, 2020).

Can Strength Training Help with Sarcopenia or Osteoporosis?

Remember that strength training can't eliminate any illness or disease, but like any other form of exercise, it can assist with your well-being. When it comes to sarcopenia or osteoporosis, strength training is beneficial and often recommended due to the ability to strengthen bone mass, muscle quality, and overall body strength. Consistent practice will simply slow down the effects of the disease.

A Fifteen-Minute Workout

This quick, fifteen-minute workout is a perfect way to introduce strength training to your exercise routine. Before you start keep the following in mind:

- Remember to warm up, dynamic stretches are advised.
- This is a rep-based workout, there is a minimum number and a maximum count, and the aim is to do better than the minimum. However, listen to your body.
- Take a minute break in between each exercise.
- Don't forget to cool down.

15 Minute Strength Training Workout

Squat with curl and knee lift

Target: Biceps, glutes, quads
- Hold both weights in each hand with your arms placed at the side of your body, lower down into a squat.
- As you rise back up lift your right knee and curl the weights to your shoulders.
- Slowly lower your weights back down to your sides and return to your squat position.
- Repeat, interchanging the knee lift, and do eight to twelve reps per side.

Shoulder overhead press

Target: Shoulders
- Place your feet hip distance apart, with weights in both hands.
- Lift your arms straight into the air, with the weights facing forward.

- As you lower them down, engage your core. Create a goal post position with your arms, where your elbows are wide, and the weights are in line with your ears.
- Return to the starting position, moving with control.
- Do eight to twelve reps.

Renegade arm row

Targets: Triceps, back, shoulders

- Put your legs together and sit back into a high squat, with your chest open and upwards.
- Slant your arms, with weights, in front of your body.
- Draw your elbows toward your hips without moving the rest of your body and return the weights to their position slowly.
- Do eight to twelve reps.

Bird dog

Target: Back, glutes, core

- Start in a tabletop position (on all fours) with your core engaged extend the right arm and left leg simultaneously.
- Hold, until your core is engaged, and return your limbs slowly before continuing to the next move.
- Do eight to ten reps per side.

Glute bridge

Targets: glutes, hamstrings

- Lie flat on your back with your knees bent and hip distance apart, you should be able to feel the back of your heels with your hands.

- Engage your core and squeeze your glutes as you lift your hips into a bridge.
- Hold and squeeze and slowly return to the starting position.
- Do eight to twelve reps.

Kneeling shoulder tap and push-up

Targets: Arms, shoulders, core

- Begin in a kneeling plank position, with your hands firmly on the ground underneath your shoulders, your back extended, and your core engaged.
- Lower down into a push-up, as close to the floor as you can get. Then push back up and with control tap your right shoulder with your left hand.
- Lower back down into a push-up, return to the plank, and tap your left shoulder with your right hand.
- Do eight to twelve push-up reps in total.

Mid back extension

Target: Back, core

- Lie face down on your mat and engage your core as you lift your abs away from the mat. Lift as high as you can, your shoulders should be moving down your back.
- Hover your upper body slightly above the ground as you lengthen your muscles, continuing to arch with muscle engagement.
- Inhale and return to the starting position.
- Do eight to twelve reps.

Full body sit up

Target: Core, shoulders, back

- Begin lying flat on the mat, with your arms extended overhead, and your legs straight and long with your feet flexed.

- Inhale and lift your arms, curling your chin into your chest, then your chest into your stomach, and exhale as your entire torso rolls up and over your legs, your arms should be reaching for your toes.

- Inhale and slowly begin to roll backward as you move through one vertebra at a time while keeping your core engaged.

- Return to the starting position with your arms over your head.

Chapter 9:
MOTIVATION AND OVERCOMING CHALLENGES

When we need to le, it is easy to lose motivation to continue, especially if we have to refocus and reconfirm the need for the choices we're making. According to Healthdirect (2022), motivation is defined as a drive that enforces and encourages us to achieve our goals. Motivation helps us to justify our actions and desires, so since one of our goals is flexibility, motivation can help us determine the reasons why we must achieve flexibility. The following questions can help you develop the motivation to achieve this goal.

- Ask yourself how much you want to achieve the goal.
- Explore what it is that you'll gain from achieving this goal.
- What are the stakes for losing and not achieving this goal?
- What are your expectations for this goal? (Healthdirect, 2022, para.1)

Ultimately, motivation serves as an unlimited resource of encouragement, it is vital because it:

- helps you solve your problems.
- helps you determine what your goals are.
- provides you with confidence and courage to change old habits.
- will gently encourage you through difficult situations. (Healthdirect, 2022)

Benefits of Motivation

There are also additional benefits to motivation, which includes:

- Developing better clarity which will help you define your goals and desires in life.
- Being able to challenge that negative voice in your head.
- Helping to increase your productivity.
- Improving your decision-making skills.
- Helping you to develop better self-control.
- Supporting you in cultivating a positive outlook on life.

How Can I Improve My Motivation?

The first step would be to acknowledge that mistakes and setbacks are natural occurrences that happen and affect our motivation levels. The next productive element would be preparation:

- Add your goal to your calendar: This will authenticate your goal and give it structure.
- Adapt this goal into a habit: Remember that habits are endurable when we're in a good and positive place.
- Plan for imperfection: Things don't always work out and sometimes you are going to stumble, so be prepared for days when you make mistakes. If you don't feel good, take a breath, and rest up.
- Set small goals to build momentum: This is the best way to trick yourself into getting back into the habit of accomplishing your goals.

- Keep track of your progress: Journaling is a great way to keep track of everything that is happening to you. It also makes you aware of your changing emotions, and possibly prepares you for burnout.

- Always reward yourself for the little wins as well as the big ones: Remember that these rewards should be equal and fair, don't reward yourself for one accomplishment more than the other.

- Embrace that negative voice in your head: Challenge it with a positive response, for every negative comment, respond with a factual positive one about yourself.

- Practice gratitude: Keep addressing those three questions in your journal.

- Boost your mood with activity: Do your best to continue your fitness levels, if it is too hard, go for a walk or stimulate your mind with an activity.

- Be mindful of your self-care practices: It is easy to forget about our overall health, so take a minute and visit your self-care pillars.

What Happens if I Lose Motivation?

Don't freak out, take a breath. Mistakes, failures, and setbacks are normal and there's no reason to slip into a negative mindset about what happened. Motivation doesn't just fade, remember that it is imbued within you because you are aware of yourself and the goals you hope to achieve. We all get demotivated sometimes and this could be due to burnout, a lack of sleep influencing your mood, or simply a lack of rest. The first thing to do when you notice that you are feeling demotivated is to breathe and find your journal—it is time to reflect on your feelings and what's happening internally. Remember that constantly challenging ourselves, particularly with activity, is going to make you feel a lot better and more confident. Here are some strategies to work through; however, not every strategy will work for you, but it is best to test them out (Morin, 2022).

- Trick your brain by acting as if you are motivated and reduce the layers of negativity in your head. You can change your behavior by actively preparing yourself for the day, showering, getting dressed, cooking a nutritional meal for breakfast, and continuing through your day. You will stumble, but through consistency, you can rebuild your motivation.

- Hit your negativity with a fact every time it begins to dismiss your ability to do anything. Every time that voice in your head tells you that you are not capable, that you are fine where you are—doing nothing—take a breath and respond with a positive fact about yourself. And if the voice in your head chooses to argue and pester you, continue with your positive remarks and argue in favor of yourself.

- Manage your to-do list realistically and figure out which of those tasks are currently non-essential. Remember the trick is to accomplish the easiest tasks on the list so that you fall into the habit of consistently completing each task.

- Focus on your self-care practices, sometimes all we need is a day of rest. On the verge of burnout, it is best to take a step back and approach the situation and everything you are feeling with honesty.

How to Overcome Challenges

Self-doubt is a major contributor to why we tend to struggle with challenges or rather why certain challenges linger as long as they do. We know that life provides challenges, and we know that the healthy thing to do is move through them, but oftentimes we find ourselves stuck within the challenge. This is due to doubt—when we begin to question ourselves, that negative voice in our head strengthens. Here are some strategies to help you through those challenges.

Make a Plan

The minute a challenging issue strikes, the natural response is to sit and wait it out while the negative voice in our heads runs free. Though we can't predict the future and plan everything, sometimes, being realistic about life and its challenges will preserve your sanity. This means acknowledging and accepting that life will throw some challenges at you and if you are not prepared for them you are going to stumble, which will require most of your strength to get back up again. So, the simplest of things to do is try and plan and aim to cultivate a more resilient mindset.

Know You Are Not Alone

Everyone struggles and everyone is aging alongside you regardless of their age. We discussed the benefits of social engagement and being in the company of other aging adults. Sometimes, the most helpful thing to do is to join a support group or reach out to trusted friends and have an honest conversation about how you are feeling.

Ask for Help

There might be a stigma attached to the aging adult asking for help from their loved ones but realistically, our bodies are changing and some of us are prone to more aches and diseases. Also, due to our declining range of mobility, the risk of falling increases each year with age. Don't feel embarrassed or believe that negative voice in your head, you are not a burden, and asking for help is perfectly acceptable. Also, when we take the step and ask for help, we're automatically acknowledging that things aren't going well for us.

Feel Your Feelings

There's nothing to gain in concealing your feelings and surely, we're too old to believe that by avoiding them we're removing them. I know that this is a strange and frightening time, and it is okay to feel any emotion you are experiencing. No one wants to grow old and have to face a decline in health, if you are upset feel it. Here's the thing, be honest about your feelings with those around you, if you feel you are struggling, let them know what you are feeling—you don't have to go into detail—and assure them that you are working on healing and accepting the situation.

Accept Support

Those around you will naturally want to help you, and though aging is a personal experience, be mindful of your words and reactions. The last thing we want to do is come across as ungrateful. If you are struggling to discuss your issue with your family and friends, therapy and group counseling sessions can be beneficial.

Help Others

Remember that each of us is going through some form of challenge, so if you recognize similar symptoms in someone close to you offer your support and assistance. Make sure not to overwhelm them and respect their boundaries.

Be Positive

Positive mindsets are a great countermeasure to combating negativity, self-doubt, and mental health issues. Cultivating positivity requires mindfulness techniques and healthy mood boosters that we get by engaging in physical exercise and social activity. Positiveness contributes wonderful benefits like increasing your lifespan and lowering the effects of mental health issues like depression and anxiety.

Never Give Up

It is very important to work on your resilience, realistically it is impossible to predict the challenges that await each of us; the closest we can get through preparation and acceptance of our situations. Giving up is the equivalent of self-doubt and will stay with you, contributing toward the negative voice in your head. A way to combat this is with productivity, sticking to your schedule every day, and holding yourself accountable while still being respectful of yourself.

Work SMART

Sometimes the simplest thing to do is redefine your purpose by writing down your goals. Revisit the SMART section.

Embrace Yourself

Learn to accept your flaws and whenever a stressful situation arises, remind yourself of your values and expectations. Remember that the challenges we face are infused with self-doubt and the most sustainable method for coping with it is by strengthening your confidence. But like any form of emotion, self-doubt is manageable.

Chapter 10:
MOVEMENT INTO DAILY LIFE

By now, we've cleared up any misconceptions about you being way too old or fragile to pursue a more active lifestyle. Cultivating a fitness routine at this stage in life can be overwhelming and even odd, but let's take the opportunity to address any questions for those of us who are struggling to adapt to flexibility. It can be a strenuous practice if you are struggling to increase mobility or constantly find yourself experiencing forms of pain. This is why it is time to discuss other ways to promote a healthy active lifestyle. So, if you are struggling to develop your flexibility, it is best to take a step back and reassess what needs to change. Breaks are important to include throughout your fitness journey since we often find ourselves aggressively launched into the mindset of achieving and accomplishing new goals, only to feel utterly defeated when we fail.

This effect is known as a plateau, and it is defined as a specific stage in your fitness journey where your body fails to improve because it is simply used to the demand of the workout. Another way of defining a plateau is viewing it as your body being bored with your current program. Experiencing a plateau is normal and a common tip is to switch up your exercise or the repetition count to avoid monotony because once your body enters this phase it won't reap any benefit from the workout. Here are some reasons why a plateau might occur:

- Your training routine has become ineffective.
- You have been overtraining.
- You are not pushing yourself enough.
- Your training schedule is inconsistent.
- You haven't provided enough recovery time.
- You are on the verge of burnout.
- Your diet and overall lifestyle are unhealthy.
- You are not sleeping well.

So, if your flexibility routine isn't working, you may have entered a plateau. Other signs of a plateau are when certain movements within your workout feel moderately easier and yet you are not improving, you are not building any muscle, or you haven't made significant progress with a particular stretch or yoga pose. Your weight and whether you have been feeling weaker after your practice are also signs to be mindful of. So, if the practice no longer feels like a challenge, you have likely hit a plateau. However, it is nothing to be concerned about, it can be resolved. Here are some strategies to help you through your plateau:

- Switch up your routine: Take a step back from what you are currently doing and try something new, and possibly different and more fun. The aim is to switch up the intensity and the duration of your workout, so if you notice that nothing is happening with yoga, maybe switch to a faster-paced style of yoga or include strength training.
- Try something new: Don't be afraid to explore, if you originally felt that weight training is not for you, give it a chance or maybe go for regular swims. A great defense against a plateau is a challenge; however, remember moderation and don't rush to end the plateau.

- Prioritize recovery and rest: It is easy to dismiss our tiredness and fatigue, or that we're on the brink of burnout. Though the plateau is naturally unwelcome it does allow us to pause and re-evaluate what exactly is happening. Also, with rest and recovery, we're focused on promoting a healthier sleep schedule because when we are overtraining our sleep gets hindered. I shouldn't have to stress this again but remember that the success of your fitness goal is contingent on your body's ability to repair itself.

There isn't an exact timeframe for a plateau to end, though usually, it can last for up to eight to twelve weeks.

Active Living Tips

Regardless of if it is a plateau or an issue with your flexibility, it is always best to be mindful and open to additional sources of activity. This means that with mindfulness common chores like sweeping the floor can become a stimulating activity. Here are some examples of how to include more activities in your daily life.

- Go for walks, not only are you stretching those muscles but if you are walking with a friend or relative, you are stimulating your mind with a positive connection.
- Join some fun local tournaments in your area, the internet is a friend in this regard, look up if any senior clubs or fun tournaments are happening:
  - This could be joining a bowling league, a bocce team, an aerobics class, a book club, or even a garden club.

- Sign up for some classes to improve your skillset:
  - This can be an art class, a woodworking class, a cooking class, or a language class.
- Dance a bit more, signing up for dance classes can be extremely fun and even sentimental:
  - I'm sure you must have been interested in learning how to tango at some point.
- Give beer pong a chance now that you are a bit older, this is going to bring back interesting memories, even if you haven't played it before I'm sure there are memories associated with the game. Now, you don't have to fill the cups with beer, it could be juice or water, the aim is simply to have some fun, revisit some old memories, and stimulate your brain health.
- Learn an instrument, maybe you have always been gifted, but I'm sure there is an instrument you haven't tried yet:
  - Drumming is a good hobby to up, it reduces stress, alleviates pain, and keeps you mentally sharp.
- Go for a swim, in fact, how do you feel about aqua aerobics, our lungs aren't what they used to be, but regular swimming or aqua aerobics is fun:
  - Swimming is regarded as a perfect exercise that actively engages the full body.

Travel Adventures

If you are an avid traveler, it is still possible to maintain your fitness goals or perhaps you have just entered retirement and pursued overall health to prepare for your travel. Regardless of your reasons for traveling, let's address some common issues that can arise with travel. Before we get to that, I'm also going to assume that you have prepared for your travels and thought I'd include a checklist for you.

CHECKLIST FOR TRAVELING

- Check in with your medical practitioner well in advance of your upcoming travel and inform them of the places you are going to visit.

- Make sure to make notes regarding any precautions you should consider.

- Now is also the time to ask any question regarding your health and travel.

- Do some research and find out if there are any vaccinations you need to have, many overseas travel destinations require this. Once you have confirmation, go and speak to your medical practitioner.

- Discuss your current medication with your medical practitioner and how a change in the time zone can affect the consumption of the medication.

- Pack your medications in your carry-on bag and make sure you have the doctor's note nearby.

- Select the aisle seat on long flights, I know everyone fusses over the window, but trust me you don't want to be that person who needs to apologize for getting up constantly to use the bathroom.

- Always print and share your travel documents with a trusted relative.

- Refuel with water and try to opt for the more nutritional snacks on the plane.

- It is okay to get up from your seat during the flight to stretch a bit, just be mindful of those around you.

- Be picky about the hotel you are going to choose, make sure that it meets your needs.
- Be mindful of how much information you are sharing about your trip on social media, thieves are known to stalk social media for potential targets.
- Always follow the public health guidelines of the other city or country you are visiting.

Staying Active on Your Travels

Despite how fun traveling excursions can be, they are stressful and can distract us from our goals. The first few days may overwhelm your system and goals, the best thing to do is be conscious that you may not meet the same goals or results as you did at home. Here are some tips:

- Go for a morning run or walk: Make sure to research the area you are staying in and try setting a specific time to hold yourself accountable for this goal.
- Be mindful of your meals: We have the habit of changing our diet when we're on vacation, so be mindful of the foods you are eating.
- It is perfectly fine to indulge a bit but be mindful of overindulging: Balance goes a long way. If you feel yourself reaching for more food or dessert, maybe get up and take a walk.
- Stay hydrated: Remember that your body needs higher levels of endurance when you travel, so rest up, drink water, and try to cut back on alcohol.
- Don't forget to take your vitamins and supplements: Strengthen your immune system, it is easy to catch the flu or a cold.

The goal should be your health, so do your best to plan and check in with your medical practitioner before your travels.

Some tips on how to maintain your fitness goals while traveling:

- Try to take the stairs where possible. Start small, if you are staying on the sixth floor start by taking the elevator up to the fourth floor and take the stairs the rest of the way.
- Opt to sightsee by walking instead of hopping into a taxi—or whichever means of transport is available—but be mindful and don't overexert yourself. Maybe plan your day-to-day with particular walkable areas in mind.
- Use the pool and enjoy yourself, remember that swimming is a great overall body workout.
- Find restaurants and cafes near your hotel or perhaps take a taxi halfway to the restaurant and walk the rest of the way—be mindful of the safety measures within the area.
- Be open to the fitness program available at the gym of your hotel.

Adventurous Experiences

We've all heard the story about those eighty to ninety-year-old people skydiving and declaring that they will return the next year if given the chance. The truth is there's no reason for you not to explore more adventures as you continue to age. However, it is best to be mindful about whether your body can endure this strain. Always check in with your medical practitioner about whether your health can endure. According to Highergrounds, being more adventurous in life offers our health extraordinary benefits it doesn't matter if the adventures are physical or mental it ultimately makes us feel good about ourselves. "It fires up the same regions of the brain that getting a reward does" (Highergrounds, 2020, para.1).

This fire or feeling motivates us to continue seeking thrilling experiences. However, remember that for some of us, a thrilling experience is the equivalent of mental challenges like puzzles. Adventurous experiences stimulate the brain and with consistent practice, your brain health will improve, this is "because you're constantly learning, which creates new synapses and strengthens existing ones, a process known as neuroplasticity, she says. This can make your brain sharper" (Highergrounds, 2020, para.1)

Benefits of Being More Adventurous

Change

Change will become easier with time and since our bodies and health are conditioned to constantly endure change, accepting change easily is a beneficial skill to develop. However, it has been noted that those who are drawn to thrilling experiences develop an impressive tolerance toward the sensations of uncertainty. This means that they can adapt to change regardless of the situation or experience. According to Hightergrounds, these people "enjoy engaging with unfamiliar things, are innately curious about the world, and creatively adapt to change instead of being fearful of it" (2020, para.2).

To nurture this quality, you must seek adventurous experiences. However, remember that these experiences don't have to be wild or extreme, the thrilling sensation we're seeking is personal—it is about you, and this could be anything, such as:

- Joining an art, ceramics, or sculpting class.
- Signing up for a language course online.
- Trying a new workout, like Pilates, barre, or adult gymnastics.

It is best to remember that seeking adventure requires you to be a bit more courageous.

Evolving

Your confidence will encourage growth which means that the more thrilling experiences you complete, the more your confidence improves. In the previous section, we discussed that one of the main skills you need to succeed at being more adventurous is courage. Many of us struggle with courage and it is because courage is such a bold sensation, it gloats with confidence, doesn't it? This is what's so great about seeking thrilling experiences, not only is it going to improve your confidence level but by doing so, you'll start to become more courageous. By consistently seeking thrilling experiences we're forcing ourselves to constantly evolve. Remember to seek the thrills that bring you joy, if you don't feel comfortable with them, there are other options, such as:

- joining a drama club or a choir
- doing improv at your local comedy club
- doing volunteer work

The goal is to challenge your comfort zone and constantly move forward.

Fluidity

So, when you are in the process of the thrilling experience, you are focused and engaged in what is happening, which is good for your brain and cognitive skills. According to Highergrounds, you then feel a pleasant sense of flow take over, "everything else except what you're concentrating on falls away, and a general sense of well-being takes over. 'You go out of time, out of yourself,' (2020, para.2). This state is referred to as an "intense feel-good state" that creates a saturating fluidity. Research focused on participants in adventure sports revealed that they were able to achieve this state. "If you looked at our brains in the flow state, you'd likely see rhythmic spikes of dopamine, which is associated with engagement and pleasure. Even better, those positive feelings can last beyond the activity itself" (Highergrounds, 2020, para.2).

Fulfillment

Feeling fulfilled is the equivalent of accomplishing a goal, it might be better because it gives off a reward kind of feeling. The research explored this phenomenon, "Adventurous people tend to have stronger feelings of satisfaction about how they're living their lives. They have a sense of flourishing" (Highergrounds, 2020, para.2). Researchers claimed that when these participants faced a challenge, regardless of its level of difficulty, they were infused with joy.

Trusting Yourself

We spoke about learning to listen to your body—you remember the mind and body connection, right, and how they positively inform one another? —and now I want to advise you to trust yourself. When it comes to trust we often only associate the sensation with other people. Trust is a bond between people, it is about displaying kindness, strength, and resilience to the other person. In return, we want to notice these attributes in the person who offers their friendship to us. Trust is also about reliability and sacredness and when this bond is damaged it negatively affects us, mentally, emotionally, and physically. However, when it comes to trusting ourselves, the feeling complicates because we're naturally harder on ourselves and way more critical.

Because we've been discussing change and the influence of confidence on courage—and vice-versa—it is interesting to note how much consistency and change rely on trust. We have to wholeheartedly trust ourselves during this changing and strange time in our lives, because not only are we aiming to improve our flexibility, but we're also trying to prevent the risk of falling. Trust is extremely important when it comes to implementing new goals and methods in our lives, you know that change portrays itself as an untrustworthy candidate. It can be as plain as saying that if you don't believe in yourself, you don't trust yourself.

Another issue with a lack of trust or broken trust, is that when we make a mistake or fail at achieving a goal, we begin to lose faith in ourselves, and this ultimately damages our motivation to continue. And let's be honest, this is a difficult experience, and we will make mistakes throughout it but if negativity imbues our mindset, removing ourselves from that bad place will be challenging and honestly easy to dismiss. Building trust with you will positively affect and influence your brain health and boost your critical thinking skills and decision-making skills. Here are some tips to help you build trust within yourself.

Be Yourself

Life has got even shorter so there's no point in wasting time trying to please other people or following any aesthetic that brings you no joy. If a situation or a person makes you feel uncomfortable or unsure about yourself and the lifestyle changes you are implementing simply walk away and distance yourself. If this person is family or the situation is a family event, space and time are good enforcers to have. This means that you always insert space between the person and yourself, and when it comes to the event limit your time there.

Set Reasonable Goals

We've already discussed the importance of being realistic and accepting of the circumstances you are in. No one wants to age, those who claim that they look forward to it are delusional, aging is terrifying and uncomfortable. But accepting this early on or constantly reminding yourself of this fact will bring you peace of mind. Failure and mistakes are bound to happen; however, they shouldn't be failing because you have been overly ambitious and disregarding the reality of the situation. Be mindful of your goals.

Always Be Kind to Yourself

We previously discussed the power of affirmation; it does go a long way in building confidence. The great thing about repetition is that the more we enforce it the easier affirmations are to believe. Journalling is a great method to build up kindness, remember that the person we tend to be the unkindest towards is ourselves. So, reflect in your journal about your fears and insecurities, but every negative thing you write about yourself must be paired with a positive attribute about yourself. The goal is to do this with your mind and that negative voice in your head, each time that voice launches at your self-esteem with a negative comment, stop it and respond with a positive comment about yourself.

Lean on Your Strengths

No one is good at everything in life. Yes, some people appear more talented, but have you taken a minute and wondered why they are good at so many things? We have the habit of naming skills as gifts people are born with, but the truth is that hard work pays off. We must constantly aim to learn and improve upon our skillset and must want to challenge ourselves. The best place to start is with your current strengths and aim at improving them. For example, if you have always been a good baker, why not sign up for a baking class and improve your current skills while learning new ones? Remember it is good to challenge yourself.

Spend Time with Yourself

We know that being alone and feeling lonely are two different emotions. We also know that aging procures high levels of loneliness and to combat this we need social engagement and activity. However, when it comes to trusting yourself, you need to feel comfortable alone because there will be moments when social engagement and activity aren't able to happen. For example, you could be ill or nursing an injury, and though loved ones may be around, the brain—its negativity—will take advantage of this and convince you that you are lonely. The trick to combating this is knowing how to be by yourself, now this doesn't mean sitting alone or watching TV alone. It is about finding joy in simply being by yourself while practicing a particular activity. This could be:

- reading a book or practicing mediation
- doing crochet or baking a treat
- taking an online class or caring for your garden

Remember that no one but you can fully comprehend yourself and the emotions present within you. Be kind to yourself.

Conclusion:
EVOKING JOY

Remember that despite this being the end of the book your journey is one of continuous progress. Society tends to present life after fifty as a journey that is or rather can only go downhill. It is strange how easy it is to believe this. We read and are told that growing older means that there is no point in continuing to live our best lives or preserving a healthy and functional life. Misconceptions about age will never fully diminish and the only sane thing to do is acknowledge the set of changes that await us and accept them. I hope that you have found comfort in the information shared in this book; however, I want to add one more thought on the sensation of joy.

Some time ago I read that the difference between happiness and joy is related to the concept of real time. Have you heard the younger folk use this phrase? It means that whatever is happening is happening now and emerged due to our relationship with the internet. Well, this article I read, though focused on ways to promote happiness in your life, actually dismissed happiness as being a lesser form of joy and as a short-lived sensation. The consensus was that happiness was only possible or able to exist after the fact, so to feel happy you must have first experienced the thing that caused the happiness. This means that we're never happy in real-time or during the moment. Another approach to the concept claims that happiness only exists after a memory has been formed and we can only relive this impression of happiness.

Do you agree with this concept? At first, I did too, but then the article introduced the sensation of joy. Joy is described as a permanent sensation that is present within us, it remains there and simply needs to be cultivated for it to positively affect our being. Joy is regarded as a more spiritual practice, though not in the strict sense, this kind of spirituality is about you. In some way, joy is related to mindfulness and teaches each of us to preserve the feelings that matter most to us. Now, I don't want to preach about getting older and tell you that there is more to life than cranky old bones. Realistically, health-related issues are going to get more difficult, but this doesn't mean that we should drift off into despair and wait for the end to arrive. Of course, not.

Joy is defined as a more wholesome emotion whereas the short-lived nature of happiness is fleeting and never present when sadness is evoked. However, joy is always with us, sometimes we forget about it, overlook it because our lives get so exhaustively busy or because we're stuck in our own minds. This means that you shouldn't chase or try to preserve happiness, instead try to cultivate joy into your life. According to Bevill and Smith (2023), when we're infused with positive emotion it improves our outlook on life and response to action, which ultimately promotes connection with our community and our sense of belonging. "When we connect with a deeper sense of meaning in our lives and contribute to creating a community that aligns with what is important in our lives, we experience a deeper sense of joy" (Bevill & Smith, 2023, para.3).

Numerous studies have explored the connection between longevity and various factors like socioeconomic status or physiological elements, that actively affect the lifespan (Bevill & Smith, 2023). Research has found that strong relationships are vital to our overall health. An impressive study observed a group of adults and their descendants for eighty-five years, "documenting a myriad of influences throughout their successes and failures. The study found that while physical health is not to be ignored, those who had strong and satisfied personal relationships were on the path to the longest lives" (Bevill and Smith, 2023, para.4). The conclusion of the study determined that "joy can be derived from the feeling of connection – or reconnection – with ourselves and others, the participants who felt strongly bonded with their loved ones showed greater signs of health and vitality than participants who reported having weaker relationships" (Beville and Smith, 2023, para.5).

It is best to remember that healthy connections with people not only protect our minds but also our bodies—the mind and body connection, remember? But since joy can declare such positive sensations within our lives, the best thing for us to do is find ways to cultivate it within our daily lives. Bevill and Smith, provide research-based suggestions for us to follow, (2023, para.6).

- Foster relationships: Building a deep and meaningful connection with people is fundamental to our lifespan. However, keep in mind that you don't have to connect with everyone you meet and sometimes it is perfectly fine to let go of certain relationships. By ensuring the health of the connection we're opening ourselves up not only to friendship but also trust. Trust can be complicated and frightening, especially since not everyone has our best interests at heart. So, be mindful of the people you are choosing to connect with, and don't feel guilty for choosing to remove some of them from your life. The aim is to maintain a healthy balance between our mind and body condition.
  - Spending time with friends and family, meeting up for coffee, going to the museum, or simply going for a walk are great little

experiences. Try to meet up with your loved ones at least once a month.

- Don't forget to practice gratitude: There is power in reflection and taking the time to actively check in with ourselves promotes optimal strength and wellness. We already discussed how journalling before bed is a great place to start, and that it is normal to feel overwhelmed by the question of three things that you are grateful for after each day. However, with consistency, you'll find yourself consciously and honestly being able to list down various little joys. Remember that like goals and accomplishments, joy also comes in all shapes and sizes.
  - Use your journal throughout the day, if you are stressed or feel upset, after you have calmed down, open up your journal to reflect on the emotions you are feeling, but remember to also visit your journal when things are going well, even if it is just a little note, write it down.

- Let go of what you can't control: Specifically, the process of growing older. For many of us, change is uncomfortable and the last thing that I want to tell you is that it is okay to feel what you feel or to get over it. We each process our emotions differently and sometimes we need help to understand what exactly we're feeling. If you feel that you are in this position, reach out to a trusted friend or relative or find a therapist to talk about your emotions. So, before you hurry to let go of difficulty, toxicity, or trauma ask yourself if it is coming from a mindful position because often, we find that our verbal declaration doesn't match our emotions. So, take your time, and when you are ready to acknowledge your feelings, you'll be able to accept the reality of the situation.

- Be honest with yourself, remember in order to accept our circumstances we must first acknowledge our feelings.

- Enjoy yourself: This one relates a bit to practicing self-compassion and though compassion is generally about understanding someone else's emotions and responding with kindness, the goal is to do this for yourself. So, think about those connections you are strengthening with your family and friends, they require respect and generosity to succeed; however, when it comes to the self, we tend to be a bit more negligent about the way we speak and treat ourselves. A great thing to do whenever you find yourself launched into a negative mindset or attack yourself is to mindfully pause and practice some yogic breathing—the three-part breathing technique works best here—and reflect.
  - Be kind and use positive affirmation daily, it might be weird at first but read an affirmation to yourself every morning or leave a kind note to yourself, especially when you are feeling a bit stressed or out of sorts.

I hope that you continue your fitness journey, remember that flexibility isn't defined overnight or over six months. It is a practice reliant on consistency, know that despite how difficult certain moments are they will pass. When we were younger the common form of encouragement expressed throughout difficulty was to look toward the future, which now might sound like a strange idea. I still can't help but wonder what exactly or how this expression works for us now that we've already entered the future. Remember to work on cultivating your joy, and always seek to find it, even when things are difficult or filled with sadness, there is always something worth being grateful for.

Again, thank you for purchasing this book. If you have found it helpful, please go to Amazon and write a brief review. This would be so appreciated and will give other seniors an idea of what this book is all about.

And please be looking for other books for seniors that we will be publishing in the very near future.

Seniors are our primary focus, and your input will be most appreciated.

Nick and Nora

REFERENCES

Bevill, L., & Smith, B. (2023, March 23). *Cultivate Joy to Improve Well-being.* IE Insights. https://www.ie.edu/insights/articles/cultivate-joy-to-improve-well-being/

Cafasso, J. (2018, July 18). *How Many Cells Are in the Human Body? Types, Production, Loss, More,* Healthline. https://www.healthline.com/health/number-of-cells-in-body

Chertoff, J. (2019, May 23). *Dynamic Stretching: Benefits, When to Use, Examples, and More,* Healthline. https://www.healthline.com/health/exercise-fitness/dynamic-stretching.

Cleveland Clinic. (2021, January 18). *Labyrinthitis: Causes, Symptoms, Treatment & What it Is.* https://my.clevelandclinic.org/health/diseases/22032-labyrinthitis

Cleveland Clinic. (2022, July 19). *What are free radicals? And why should you care?* https://health.clevelandclinic.org/free-radicals/

Cleveland Clinic. (2023, September 6). *The Health Benefits of Tai Chi.* https://health.clevelandclinic.org/the-health-benefits-of-tai-chi/

Culpepper Place. (2019, June 4). *Answering Your Questions About Exercise for Seniors.* https://culpepperplaceassistedliving.com/exercise-for-seniors/

Davidson, K. (2021, September 20). *The Definitive Guide to Healthy Eating in Your 50s and 60s.* Healthline. https://www.healthline.com/nutrition/healthy-eating-50s-60s

Elridge, L. (2022, October 12). *Free radicals: definition, cause, and role in cancer.* Verywell Health. https://www.verywellhealth.com/information-about-free-radicals-224103

Esthetic Center. (n.d.). *Intrinsic Vs. Extrinsic Skin Aging - What's The Difference?* https://www.estheticscenter.com/blog/intrinsicvsextrinsicaging

Gould, W. R. (2021, March 21). *What Is Tai Chi?* Verywell Mind. https://www.verywellmind.com/what-is-tai-chi-5073074

Hart, P. (n.d.). *What Is the Mind-Body Connection?* University of Minnesota. https://www.takingcharge.csh.umn.edu/what-is-the-mind-body-connection

Healthdirect. (2022, October 19). *Motivation: How to get started and staying motivated.* https://www.healthdirect.gov.au/motivation-how-to-get-started-and-staying-motivated

Highergrounds. (2020, August 4). *The Health Benefits of Being Adventurous, According to Psychologists.* https://www.highergroundsmgmt.com/post/the-health-benefits-of-being-adventurous-according-to-psychologists

Hoshaw, C. (2022, March 29). *What Mindfulness Really Means and How to Practice.* Healthline. https://www.healthline.com/health/mind-body/what-is-mindfulness

Lam, P. (n.d.). *What is Tai Chi & what are the health benefits? (complete guide).* Tai Chi for Health Institute. https://taichiforhealthinstitute.org/what-is-tai-chi/

Madison. (2021, January 18). *How To Manage Balance Problems In Seniors.* MeetCaregivers. https://meetcaregivers.com/balance-problems-in-seniors/

McCoy, J. (2021, November 13). *An Upper-Body Warm-Up to Prep Your Back, Shoulders, and Chest for Action.* SELF. https://www.self.com/gallery/upper-body-warm-up

MedlinePlus. (2021, February 22). *What is a cell?* https://medlineplus.gov/genetics/understanding/basics/cell/

Mind Tools. (n.d.). *SMART Goals.* https://www.mindtools.com/a4wo118/smart-goals

Morin, A. (2022, May 23). *The Best Way to Boost Your Motivation When You Just Aren't Feeling It.* Verywell Mind. https://www.verywellmind.com/what-to-do-when-you-have-no-motivation-4796954

Pennant Hills Physiotherapy. (2022, October 7). *The Importance of Balance and How to Improve It.* WPH Physio. https://wphphysio.com.au/sports-physiotherapy-treatment/importance-balanced/

Physio-pedia. (n.d.). *Psychological Factors in Ageing.* https://www.physio-pedia.com/Psychological_Factors_in_Ageing

Preiato, D. (2021, March 24). *Active Stretching: What It Is, Benefits, and How to Do It.* Healthline. https://www.healthline.com/nutrition/active-stretching#examples

Smith, M., Segal, J., & White, M. (2023, November 8). *Staying healthy as you age.* HelpGuide.org. https://www.helpguide.org/articles/alzheimers-dementia-aging/staying-healthy-as-you-age.htm

Sportsspt. (2020, May 19). *Strength Training for Seniors: Expert Advice to Get Started.* Optimal Sports Physical Therapy. https://optimalsportspt.com/strength-training-for-seniors/

Stefanacci, R. (2022, September). *Changes in the Body With Aging.* MSD Manuals. https://www.msdmanuals.com/home/older-people's-health-issues/the-aging-body/changes-in-the-body-with-aging

Sullivan Killroy, D. (2014, September 8). *Exercise Plan for Seniors.* Healthline. https://www.healthline.com/health/everyday-fitness/senior-workouts

Vann, M. (2016, August 1). *The 15 Most Common Health Concerns for Seniors.* EverydayHealth.com. https://www.everydayhealth.com/news/most-common-health-concerns-seniors/

Made in the USA
Las Vegas, NV
04 February 2024

85310994R00083